ORLEAN PUCKETT:
THE LIFE OF A
MOUNTAIN MIDWIFE
1844-1939

BY

KAREN CECIL SMITH

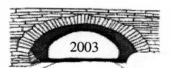

2003

Parkway Publishers
Boone, North Car...

D1410018

Copyright © 2003 by Karen Cecil Smith

Available from:

Parkway Publishers, Inc.
P. O. Box 3678
Boone, North Carolina 28607
Telephone/Facsimile: (828) 265-3993
www.parkwaypublishers.com

Library of Congress Cataloging-in-Publication Data

Smith, Karen Cecil.
   Orlean Puckett : the life of a mountain midwife, 1844-1939 /
by Karen Cecil Smith.
   p. cm.
Includes bibliographical references.
ISBN 1-887905-72-3
   1. Puckett, Orlean, 1837-1939 2. Midwives--Virginia--
Biography. I. Title.
RG950.P83 S656 2003
618.2'0092--dc21

2002155003

Editing, Layout and Book Design: Julie Shissler
Cover and Graphic Design: Aaron Burleson

CONTENTS

*In memory of Orlean Puckett
and all the dedicated women before her
who forged a path
for future generations
of midwives*

Foreword

The name of Orlean Puckett is known to the millions of visitors who stop at the Puckett cabin on the Blue Ridge Parkway in Carroll County, Virginia. The sign erected by the National Park Service provides a glimpse into her life, but the real Orlean Puckett, wife, mother and mountain midwife, is not shown.

Known to local people as "Aunt Orlean," she is famous for having birthed and lost 24 children of her own and then becoming a midwife who delivered a thousand or more babies in this mountain region of Virginia. Stories about Aunt Orlean have been handed down orally in her family and community, but this is the first book written about this remarkable woman and her life. It is a story that needs to be preserved through the written word.

A distance of time and lack of written records present a challenge in any research project. It must be remembered that by 1976 when the first interviews were conducted, nearly 40 years had passed since the death of Orlean Puckett and about 65 years since the death of her husband John. If her last child was born in 1881, 95 years separated that event and the retelling of these stories.

Through conducting her own interviews of Aunt Orlean's relatives and neighbors and using those conducted in 1976 by the Parkway seasonal interpreter, Karen Cecil Smith has been successful in recreating a picture of this incredible midwife.

Through her marriage to John Puckett, Orlean was my great, great, great aunt. The people of this book are my kinfolk and my neighbors; and the places are my community. I am proud to be a part of this family, this tradition, and this place. I am grateful to Karen Cecil Smith for telling Aunt Orlean's story.

Hillsville, VA, 2002
Shelby Inscore Puckett

Preface

For many years I have traveled from my Winston-Salem, North Carolina home to visit the beautiful Virginia mountains. The one hour drive takes me through the outskirts of Andy Griffith's Mount Airy hometown and past countless produce stands laden with mountain grown apples, peaches, cabbages, peanuts, sourwood honey, and sulfur-free molasses. Across the Virginia State line, stores that display "lottery tickets sold here" signs are framed with rows of muslin bags containing sugar cured Virginia hams.

As I head up the mountain that leads to the Parkway, my ears pop and crackle from the rising altitude. Once on the Parkway, headed east, a peace surrounds me and I feel as close to God as I could ever hope to get while on this earth. Scattered along the way are quaint but lovely churches that were rocked by mountain preacher Bob Childress. A stop at Doe Run Lodge for lunch and a climb up the tower at Groundhog Mountain are routines that mark my way. Past Mayberry Trading Post, and the small Meadows of Dan community, my journey ends at Mabry Mill where I take a moment to watch the water wheel turn and smell the acrid smoke rising from the blacksmith shop.

On the return trip west I am drawn, as always, to Milepost 189.9 and "the cabin home" of midwife Orlean Puckett. My intrigue with this midwife began when I saw the first sign that was posted in front of the crude log dwelling. Erected by the National Park Service, the sign read:

> *This was the cabin home of Mrs. Orlean Hawks Puckett from 1865 until her death in 1939 at the age of 102 years. While "Aunt Arlene" carried her skill as a midwife over trails to hundreds of mountain cabins, none of her own twenty-four children lived beyond infancy.*

I longed to learn more about this incredible woman. My research, which led me to various libraries, seemed futile for all I could find were brochures and articles that conveyed the same general information listed on the National Park Service plaque. Accepting defeat, I put all thoughts of Orlean Puckett out of my head.

It was not until another trip to the Parkway in 1997 that my interest was again ignited. What I discovered in front of the cabin was a new, more detailed sign. This one read:

> *Born in 1837, "Aunt" Orelena Hawks Puckett lived here during the latter of her 102 years. She was often heard to say, "The forest was green when I was a-born and I'm green yet." A bride at 16, Mrs. Puckett and her husband first farmed below nearby Groundhog Mountain. Mrs. Puckett was past age 50 when she began a long career of midwifery. She assisted at the births of more than 1,000 babies, delivering the last in 1939, the year she died. It has been said she never lost a child or mother through her own fault. Ironically, none of Mrs. Puckett's own 24 children lived beyond infancy. Regardless of weather, "Aunt" Orelena went wherever and whenever called. Sometimes on horseback, often walking, the midwife brought assurance and kindness to all she visited. When she began her practice around 1890 her fee was one dollar, and "when times was good," six dollars. Often receiving food or other goods in lieu of money, she generously shared all she had with neighbors or those in need. Today, Orelena Puckett is remembered in this area for her witty, cheerful personality, as well as for her unselfish and skillful practice as a midwife.*

A picture was included on the plaque that showed the midwife seated in front of the cabin, holding the last baby she delivered. As I gazed onto the aged face of Orlean Puckett, I knew that I had to know more about her. On that quiet, mild, spring day, surrounded by split rail fences, mountain laurel and purple larkspur, I was convinced there was a story that needed to be told, and I wanted to be the one to tell it.

More determined than I had been the first time, my research began with a phone call to the historical society in Stuart, Virginia. Although I was not able to obtain any information at that time, my inquiry eventually brought about a response from one of Orlean Puckett's relatives. Shelby Puckett, an educator and member of the Carroll County Historical Society, called to tell me that she was related to Orlean and John Puckett and that her husband Raleigh was also a relative of theirs. Shelby was eager to share information about her distant relative and invited me to her home just off the Virginia Parkway.

That day marked the beginning of almost three years of research on the life of Orlean Puckett. Although I scoured through court records, genealogies, newspapers, census reports, land deeds, and other vital records, the majority of the information I obtained was an oral history, relayed by the midwife's many relatives, friends, and neighbors. Without the help of Shelby and Raleigh Puckett, who introduced me to those individuals, this book would not be possible.

Most of the people I spoke with, some in their 70s, 80s, and 90s, were delivered by Orlean Puckett. Sadly, a few of them have died since my research began. The comment that echoed throughout my interviews with those individuals was "please tell the true story."

I have striven to do so in this book, which is my tribute to the life of a remarkable mountain midwife who gained the love and respect of so many individuals along Virginia's Blue Ridge Parkway.

Winston-Salem, North Carolina
Karen Cecil Smith

Acknowledgements

I would like to offer thanks to several people for their encouragement and support during the five years it took to create this book. They have been steadfast in their belief of this project. My husband, George Stanley Smith, never doubted my writing ability and was always respectful of my creative time and space. My mother, Delila Johnson Cecil, accompanied me on most of my interviews and asked the questions that I didn't. She read my manuscript several times, offered advice, and was my biggest cheerleader. Phyllis Roberson Hoots, educator, historian, and dear friend, helped greatly with the editing and prodded me along when I was discouraged. Shelby Inscore Puckett spent many hours collecting information, provided answers to my questions, and attended most of the interviews.

Finally, I would like to thank all of the Virginia mountain people who welcomed me into their homes and shared their remembrances of Orlean Puckett. Special thanks also to Wavy Worrell, Shelby Puckett, Raleigh Puckett, Tracey Puckett Stump, and Marvin Hawks for the wonderful family photographs they provided.

April 15, 2002
Karen Cecil Smith
North Carolina

Interviews of the following individuals contributed greatly to the creation of this book. Their relationship to Orlean Puckett is listed below:

Mr. Ellis Bowman (deceased)[1]	Neighbor
Nannie Bowman (deceased)[3]	Neighbor
Owen Bowman[3]	Neighbor
Mrs. Fannie Brady (deceased)[1]	Neighbor
Dewey Culler (deceased)[1]	Neighbor
Foy Hawks[3]	Great Grandnephew
Marvin Hawks[3]	Great Grandnephew
Lottie Marshall[3]	Great Grandniece
Mr. and Mrs. Coy Martin (deceased)[1]	Neighbors
Mr. Lackie Pruitt (deceased)[1]	Neighbor
Mr. Raymond Pruitt (deceased)[2]	Neighbor
Mrs. Raymond Pruitt (deceased)[1]	Neighbor
Mrs. Bell Puckett (deceased)[1]	Neighbor
David Puckett[3]	Great-Great Grandnephew
Hattie Puckett[2]	Great Grandniece
Larma Puckett[2]	Great Grandniece
Libby Puckett[2]	Great Grandniece
Raleigh Puckett[3]	Great Grandnephew
Shelby Puckett[3]	Great-Great Grandniece
Erby Quesinberry (deceased)[1]	Husband of Iduna
Iduna Quesinberry (deceased)[2]	Great Niece
Dee Spellings[3]	Great Grandniece
Icy Vass[3]	Great Grandniece
Ninevah Willis (deceased)[3]	Neighbor
Wavy Worrell[2]	Great Grandniece
Wade Worrell[3]	Great-Great Grandnephew

[1]*Interviewed in 1976 by Brenda Bowers, Seasonal Naturalist at Mabry Mill.*
[2]*Interviewed by both Brenda Bowers and Karen Cecil Smith.*
[3]*Interviewed by Karen Cecil Smith.*

Chapter 1
The Early Years

"The forest was green when I was a-born and I'm green yet."
Orlean Hawks Puckett

For over one hundred years a veil of mystery has shrouded the memory of midwife Orlean Hawks Puckett. Known to many along Virginia's Blue Ridge Mountains as a loving, selfless woman who successfully birthed over a thousand babies, she was accused by some of murdering her own 24 children. Those individuals who did not place the blame directly on Orlean were quick to point their finger at her husband John, a hardy mountain man who was reputed to have a fondness for the devil's brew.

To this day the controversy over the true story of Orlean Puckett continues. Twenty-six graves scattered in family cemeteries just off the Blue Ridge Parkway and a monument that honors the mountain midwife are not the only visible reminders of her life. The offspring of five generations of babies she delivered continues to populate the Virginia counties of Patrick and Carroll and spread onward into other states. Those generations carry with them and pass on to future generations memories of a midwife they called Aunt Orlean.

Aunt Orlean's beginnings were humble. As Ninevah Willis, a retired Carroll County educator and author who knew her, remarked, "It is interesting that one little old woman could leave behind so much history that involves so many people."

Orlean Puckett was born in 1844 in a small Virginia mountain community today known as Lambsburg. A secluded oasis that reaches out to touch the North Carolina state line, Lambsburg is framed by the majestic Blue Ridge Mountains on the north, Fisher Peak on the west, and Sugar Loaf Mountain on the east.

Originally called Rocksburg, because of the many mountain rocks that tumbled down to rest in its valley, the area was later named

Lambsburg in honor of Jehu Carmen Lamb, a gunsmith who manufactured guns for the Confederate Army at his factory on Flat Branch. Lamb settled in Rocksburg in 1860 and was instrumental in the development of the community. The first post office, in which Lamb's daughter Mariam served as postmistress, was established in 1866.[1]

Aside from its natural aesthetics, Rocksburg possessed utilitarian components that no doubt appealed to the early settlers. Unlike some of its neighboring Carroll County communities, Rocksburg provided level stretches of land ideal for planting, cultivating, and harvesting crops. Stewarts, Pauls, and Elk Creeks furnished crystal clear water for both man and beast, as well as food for a hungry mountain family.

Perhaps Rocksburg's greatest attraction was its close proximity to the large trading center of Mount Airy, North Carolina. From Rocksburg, mountaineers could easily herd their animals a few miles to market and sell or barter bushels of newly gathered chestnuts, blackberries, cherries, peaches, and apples. Sourwood honey, sorghum molasses, and cabbages would have been, as they are today, items sought after by flatlanders.

Given all these amenities, it is easy to understand why Orlean Puckett's grandfather Abraham Hawks purchased land in the Rocksburg area. In 1801 Abraham acquired 344 acres on the head waters of Pauls Creek and in 1802 added to his holdings an additional 43 acres on Stewarts Creek. Seven years later he purchased land on Elk Creek, which increased his holdings in Rocksburg to 418 acres.

Hardin Hawks, Abraham's second born son and Orlean's father, most likely acquired some of that land after his marriage on October 31, 1836. At the age of 21, Hardin married Matilda Puckett, an 18-year-old from neighboring Grayson County, Virginia. The two set up housekeeping in a small log cabin along the shores of Stewarts Creek in close proximity to Abraham and his wife Elizabeth.

In those days, men tilled the land on the homestead, most likely planting typical mountain crops of corn, cabbages, beans, and potatoes. Like his fellow mountaineers, Hardin probably hunted deer, wild turkey, ruffed grouse, squirrel, rabbit, and the occasional groundhog. Quiet afternoons would have been spent on the banks of Stewarts Creek, fishing for trout and relaxing with a draught of locally made corn whiskey.

While Hardin performed "man's work," Matilda, like most mountain wives, would have tended to the ordinary affairs of housekeeping, such as cooking, cleaning, making lye soap, patching quilts, sewing clothes, milking the cow, feeding the chickens, and gathering eggs. Harvesting vegetables, fruit, nuts, and berries was also in the realm of "woman's work."

Most mountain farms abounded with fruit trees and wild blackberry vines. During that period, ripe chestnuts, a mainstay for mountain families and foraging hogs, covered forest floors in autumn. On cold winter nights, the sweet nuts were roasted in the fireplace and eaten while still warm.

According to Wavy Worrell, a great grandniece of Orlean Puckett, the Hawks family had a special recipe for chestnut stuffing:

> *Aunt Orlean stuffed her turkey with chestnuts. She'd boil and peel 'em, cook 'em in salt water and mix in breadcrumbs, onion, and salted butter. They had a chestnut orchard and there were plenty of chestnuts for roastin' and eatin', but mostly for barterin' at the store.*[2]

Chestnut leaves were also important. Made into a broth, the leaves held medicinal properties that helped in the treatment of chest colds and coughs. Sheep, that produced wool for spinning and eventually became meat for the table, grazed on lush meadow grasses. Gums, made from twenty-four to thirty-inch long sections of hollow black gum trees, drew bees that provided honey for sweetening pies and cakes. Beeswax served as a coating for thread used in quilting, sewing clothes, and making shoes. Gums were also used as rabbit traps.

Nature's bounty offered most mountain families a rich, self-sufficient lifestyle. Lots of children in a family only added to such a lifestyle and made the workload easier.

In her book *Country Living*, Ninevah Willis recorded an interview with Reverend Bob Childress, the Virginia mountain preacher who was delivered by Aunt Orlean, who encased six churches in rock along the Blue Ridge Parkway and tamed the wild men of Buffalo Mountain. Childress was also the inspiration for another book entitled *The Man Who Moved a Mountain*, written by Richard C. Davids. In Willis' book she quotes Childress as saying,

> *A man needed his 'younguns' to help in the fields or in the home. Large families were the style. They married young, so they would have time to raise large families. A family without at least eight or ten children was considered very small, indeed. The largest family I ever heard of had thirty-five children.*
>
> *The second largest family I heard of belonged to Johnny White, he had twenty-six children. In those days there was little passing [traffic] and all the children would crowd around the doors and windows and stare at the passers. One day a man drove up in his buggy, drew rein, and called out, "Hello, there." Mrs. White went out to see what he wanted, with all her twenty-six children following close behind. The man, not being used to mountain ways, tipped his hat and said, "I'm sorry I broke up your school."*
>
> *Another mountain woman went to Hillsville, the county seat, which, after all, was a small village and many miles from her home. As this was her first trip to "town" she took along all twenty-two children. She met up with a man who became annoyed as he tried to pass them on the muddy street. He spoke and said, "Are these all yours, or is it a picnic?" With arms akimbo [stretched forth], she spat back*

at him, "*I'll have you know they're all mine, and it ain't no picnic*".[3]

The size of Hardin and Matilda's family would have been considered average by mountain terms. It was not until their third year of marriage that Matilda became pregnant with their first child, Dickerson. A long span of three years followed before the next child, son William, was born. Then, in 1844, their first daughter, Orlean, was added to the Hawks family. During the years that followed, Matilda gave birth to Zachary, Andrew, Andy, J.A., Matilda, and Frances.

After she grew old, Aunt Orlean confided to friends and family that she couldn't remember the year she was born. She did, however, remember that the month was June. Wavy Worrell relayed a conversation she had with Aunt Orlean about her age:

> *She didn't know her birth date. When they were living over in Lambsburg their house burned down and the Bible got burnt up. That's where they wrote down birth dates, you know. She'd say she didn't know the date, but that 'The forest was green when I was a-born and I'm green yet'.*[4]

There has been much dispute over Orlean Puckett's birth date. A sign along Blue Ridge Parkway Milepost 189.9 states that she was "Born in 1837." Her tombstone, most likely erected by her nephew Coy Hawks, gives the date of 1839 as the year she was born.

Mrs. Ellis Bowman, a neighbor of Aunt Orlean's who was interviewed in 1976 said:

> *She looked old as far back as I can remember. She looked the same. She didn't seem to get any older, but some folks might consider that she looked a hundred. Some claim that she was 100, but I never did say nothin' about it, but I didn't believe it. Sometime in her life their property got burned and destroyed their Bible [and] birth certificates. She could remember what month she*

was born, but she didn't remember the date. She'd always say, if anybody asked her when she was born, she was born when the timber was green and she'd laugh about it. It's sometime in June she said that her birthday was. He [John Puckett] was born 1838 and she was born 1845. She said that he was seven years older than she was. Well, you might figure it and you will see yourself how old the age she was at the time she lived here.[5]

Bible entries would have been the only birth record for the older Hawks children, since birth certificates were not issued in Virginia until 1853. However, two census records confirm that the year of Orlean's birth was 1844. At the time of the 1850 Surry County Census Records, she was identified as being six years old. Interestingly, it was also noted that her little brother Zachary, four years old at the time, possessed 24 fingers and toes. Hardin was listed as a 35-year-old laborer and Matilda's age was given as 32.

In the early part of 1860, just before her marriage to John Puckett, Orlean was still living with Hardin and Matilda, as were her three younger brothers and two younger sisters. Surry County Census Records indicate that at that time she was 16 years old.

Further evidence that 1844 is a more realistic birth date comes from an article that appeared in the September 6, 1900 issue of *The Republican* newspaper. The article quoted a letter written by Reverend C. C. Haymore. In his letter Haymore wrote, "In conversation with Mrs. Puckett, she told me that she was 55 years old."[6]

Another controversy has been over the spelling and pronunciation of her name. Some called her Arlene, while others referred to her as Orelena or Aulene. Public records have named her Pauline, Alena, Aulena, Aulina, Olenah, and Llena. To family members and close friends, she was always Aunt Orlean. Great grandnephew Marvin Hawks, whose family lived with her when he was a child, confirmed that "Orlean is the correct spelling of her name."[7]

Mrs. Coy Martin, a neighbor of Orlean Puckett, who was interviewed on July 13, 1976 said, "She was known by Aunt Orlean, but no relation whatsoever to a lot of us, you know, that called her that."[8]

For the most part, Orlean Puckett was uneducated. However, several family members and friends remember her as being an intelligent woman, despite the fact that she could not read or write. Wavy Worrell recalled a conversation with Orlean regarding her short time in school:

> *She told me that she went to school maybe three days and couldn't or wouldn't say "A" when the teacher called on her. Said he whooped her and whooped her hard and she didn't go back..*[9]

While Worrell declared that Orlean knew how to write her name in full, great grandniece Larma Puckett believed she used an "X" as her signature.

Larma and her parents lived with Aunt Orlean for almost 15 years. During that period of time, Larma's mother, Rebecca, became ill and died. Larma, who was very close to Orlean, remembered her fondly as a giving and independent woman.

According to neighbor Mrs. Ellis Bowman, Orlean had enough education to know how to count money. This would have been a necessity when she made transactions at the local stores. While she mainly bartered for goods, she occasionally dealt in cash.

While Orlean Puckett may have never received a formal education, those who knew her said that she possessed a large dose of common sense, a flair for humor, and a strong ambition. There is little doubt that those traits helped her through many trials and served her well throughout her married life and midwifery career.

Chapter 2
Young Love and the Civil War

"I shall sit in the window when summer is lying
Out over the fields, and the honey-bee's hum
Lulls the rose at the porch from her tremulous sighing,
And watch for the face of my darling to come."

from the poem "Enlisted Today"
—Author Anonymous

Twenty-three miles away from Orlean Hawks' Rocksburg home in a place called Renfro Ridge, a spur of the Blue Ridge Mountains, lived a young man named John Puckett. With a birth date of June 9, 1838, John was the ninth of fifteen children born to Jacob and Sarah 'Sally' Marshall Puckett.

May Belle Smith, the author of the book *The Puckett Family,* wrote that the Pucketts were of English ancestry. They had strong ties to the Church of England. Because of their affiliation with the Crown, the Pucketts were granted land in America. They must have been motivated by dreams of adventure, not by religious restrictions or political dissent, to uproot their families and move to another country. Smith identified them as being "Soldiers of Fortune" or "Soldiers of the Crown."

Smith noted that, according to Patrick County Deed Records, Jacob Puckett purchased 245 acres of land on Renfro's Ridge on July 1, 1851. After observation of the old Puckett home place, she concluded:

There are still signs of some rocks from the chimney of the Jacob and Sarah Puckett home, located below the crest of the mountain and north of the Higher Ground Church Camp. Libby and Hattie Puckett, great-great granddaughters of Jacob and Sarah Marshall Puckett, live a few hundred yards from the old home place. The family

*cemetery is located a short distance west of the Jacob
and Sarah Puckett home."[1]*

There has been some speculation as to where John and Orlean
first met one another. David Puckett, great-great grandnephew of John
Puckett, believes that they became acquainted at a church gathering.

> *If John and Orlean didn't meet at a church
> gathering, they probably met while visiting relatives.
> Someone even said they met in a chestnut orchard.
> But church is where most of the courting took place.
> It was the only place you couldn't offend anybody.
> Primitive Baptists had what they called Fall Meetings
> or Brush Arbor, where land was cleared and visiting
> preachers spoke. People came from all over for the
> all-day meetings. Young men who didn't even attend
> church would ask to escort the girls to and from
> church, which was a form of courting.*
>
> *One time my grandfather Arthur asked a
> woman if he could escort her daughters to church.
> He'd been drinking and she could smell the liquor
> on his breath. She told him no. That really made
> him mad! He and his friends took a footbridge [a
> log that served as a bridge] that they knew the woman
> and her daughters would have to cross to get to
> and from church and cut it almost in half, then put it
> back over the creek. When the mother and her
> daughters reached the footbridge and proceeded
> to cross it, it broke in two and they tumbled into the
> creek.[2]*

Ninevah Willis quoted Reverend Bob Childress' description of
mountain courtship:

> *The courting was done without any privacy.
> There was usually only one room in the house in
> which to entertain company and also for family use.*

So, the boy would come to see the girl and sit by her, sometimes holding her hand, in the presence of her father and mother and all the other children. On one occasion the boy was very much embarrassed because there was so much he felt and so much he couldn't find the words nor the courage to say in the presence of all the family, so he sat and worried and fretted because he couldn't speak. Before he left, (just before they called 'bedtime') he finally got up enough courage to blurt out, "They just wasted purty on you when they made you, didn't they? They made you as purty as they could and then pitched a shovel full in your face."

With that breathtaking speech, he fell out of the door. They were married the next Sunday.

The only place for young people to go was to church, and there was no way to go but on a horse. Many romances blossomed and faded to and from the meeting.[3]

Childress failed to mention other community gatherings that would have provided opportunities for young men and women to get together. Neighborhood corn shuckings, pea thrashings, house raisings and wood gettings may have meant hard work, but they were a way of socializing in many mountain neighborhoods.

At corn shuckings, the corn was piled into a heap in the barnyard. Sometimes a jug of whiskey was buried in the middle of the pile. Neighbors gathered round and, after much shucking, the jug was eventually uncovered and enjoyed by the men.

Those who were fortunate enough to find a red ear of corn in the pile got to kiss the boy or girl of their choice. Sometimes other prizes, such as money or livestock, were offered to the one who held the red ear.

Although no one knows for sure how John and Orlean got together, the two started courting sometime prior to June 1860. John would have been almost 22 years old at that time and, according to Hattie Puckett, Orlean would have been six years younger.

Hattie explained that John rode his horse to Lambsburg to court Orlean, who was his third cousin.[4]

However, David Puckett argued that John and Orlean were not cousins and said that Orlean was an "import."[5]

Raymond Pruitt, who lived down the Parkway from Aunt Orlean, called the Puckett men "purebloods." He described John as slim, which he thought was a rare quality for a Puckett man.[6]

By most accounts, the young Orlean Hawks was also slim. Mrs. Raymond Pruitt recalled Orlean as a "tall, slender woman."[7]

According to Wavy Worrell, Orlean's eyes were blue and her hair was blonde:

> It was blonde during her younger days. She told me it used to be yellow. I used to comb her hair and she'd go to sleep right nearly every time. She'd say, "Well jus' scratch some dandruff off my head." And in just a little bit, why she'd be asleep and I'd get so tired. She had the most beautiful hair. It was thin then, white and as fine as silk and she wore it in a bun. I was about 10 years old. Aunt Orlean had blue eyes and one eye crossed inward.[8]

Neighbors and relatives agreed that Orlean had a defective eye. Mrs. Raymond Pruitt described it as the "worst I ever seen." Orlean's eye was also internally flawed, for she suffered from nearsightedness. As she grew older, her vision worsened.[9]

Despite her crossed eye, neighbors Lackie Pruitt and Mrs. Raymond Pruitt remembered Orlean as being attractive and nice looking.[10]

In their early years, John and Orlean would have made a striking couple. It is most likely that, true to mountain tradition, their courtship was short.

Sometime before the two married, Orlean Puckett had an experience that forever remained in her memory. Years later, she often reminisced about her adventure. Wavy Worrell recalled Aunt Orlean's tale:

> One time, I don't know where she was livin', a bunch of colored men got after her. She was carrying dinner to her daddy and brother. Had a basket full of food and she was on the footbridge and one would get on one end of the bridge and one on the other. They were after her food. Liked to scared her to death. She went hollerin' and when she got to her daddy and brother she couldn't speak to them. And usually she'd go and whistle for her daddy and brother, but she said they scared the whistle out of her. When she finally told them what had happened, they quit work and went to hunt them. Don't think they ever found them.[11]

On that day when Orlean was carrying the noontime meal to her daddy and brother, there is likelihood that the men she encountered were hungry runaway slaves who meant her no harm.

Orlean's frightening experience on the footbridge occurred in either the late spring or early summer of 1860.

The 1860 Virginia Census gives a figure of 490,865 slaves in the state of Virginia. The free colored population was listed as 58,042. In Carroll County, where Orlean Puckett lived, there were 262 slaves and 31 free colored. In neighboring Patrick County the numbers were much larger, with 2,070 slaves and 131 free colored.

According to the 1860 Patrick County Census, John was no longer living with his parents. The census entry describes Jacob Puckett as being a 61-year-old farmer. Wife Sarah was 52 years old at the time.

Seven other individuals were listed as living in the home: Hosea, age 18; Emberzetta, age 16; Ephraim, age 14; Jacob, age 12; Jubel, age 9; Churchill, a 27-year-old shoe and bootmaker; and Julia A., age 22. Churchill was John's older brother. After they married, he and his wife Julia lived with John and Sarah.

Three other married brothers are found on the 1860 Census. They are: Riley and his wife Matilda and their two children, Adam and Roda; Elijah and his wife Sally and their four children; and Doctor Floyd and his wife Elizabeth "Aunt Betty" and their three children.

"She [Aunt Orlean] married John Puckett when she was 16 years old," said Wavy Worrell, who went on to explain that "Lots of young girls were marrying then because their beaus were goin' off to be in the Civil War."[12]

After the two married, they set up housekeeping near John's parents. "Aunt Orlean and her husband first lived at the bottom of the mountain [Groundhog Mountain] in a cabin that had a lean-to," remarked Foy Hawks, great grandnephew of John and Orlean.[13] A picture of what some believed to be John and Orlean's first home shows a rustic cabin, void of chinking, that resembles a corncrib. Whether or not this was their home, Wavy Worrell confirmed that the cabin had only one room and its location at the foot of the mountain was called "The Hollow."[14]

Hattie Puckett remembered the cabin John and Orlean moved into after they married and said that the "rocks are still there, but the cabin's gone. In the 1920s there was a flood at the bottom of the mountain [where Orlean once lived]."[15]

In May of 1861, almost a year after they married and moved into their new home in The Hollow, now known as Ararat, Orlean became pregnant with daughter Julia. Earlier that same year, on April 12, Confederates under the command of General Pierre Beauregard opened fire with 50 cannons upon Fort Sumter in Charleston, South Carolina. The Civil War had begun.[16]

During his campaign for President, Abraham Lincoln voiced a public stand against slavery. One of his slogans during the 1860 Republican presidential campaign was "Millions for freedom, not one cent for slavery."[17] This meant little to the majority of mountaineers in southwestern Virginia who didn't own slaves. Surviving bitter winters, feeding their families, and struggling to maintain a self-sufficient lifestyle took precedence over the slavery issue.

However, the lure of faraway places and the thrill of adventure acted as a magnet, drawing some mountain men who had never traveled beyond the hills into the terrible conflict. Romance, too, was often involved, since many married quickly before going off to war:

> *The women throughout the South were very enthusiastic. They urged their men to join the army. Many commitments were made between the belles and their beaus. Long good-byes were said; the trains smoked and puffed as they moved the men east. Everyone knew that if war really did come it would be a short glorious affair, that these green mountain boys were the new revolutionary heroes. Very few could resist this call to arms and glory.*[18]

Others enlisted in an effort to defend their homes and way of life from Northern invasion. Confederate President Davis' call for volunteers prompted feelings of patriotism. A notice in Staunton, Virginia further ignited those feelings. It read: "Men of Virginia, To the Rescue!"[19]

For whatever reasons, John Puckett was among some of the first to enlist in Virginia. Perhaps unaware of his wife's pregnancy, he, along with his brothers, enrolled in the month of June, 1861.

John enrolled in the army at either the Patrick County, Virginia seat, which is today called Stuart, or at Wytheville. Company K, appropriately nicknamed the "Patrick County Boys," was formed in May 1861. Some of its earliest enrollments took place in Stuart, named after famed Confederate hero Major General J.E.B. Stuart.

On July 25, the unit which was in Wytheville, Virginia had grown to a compliment of four officers and 102 enlisted men. Disease depleted the strength of the company which did not leave Wytheville until August 12. At that time Company K rejoined the regiment in time to participate in the battle at Cross Lanes, West Virginia on August 26. A reorganization took place on May 12, 1862. There was a brief period when this company was detached and fought near Princeton, West Virginia on May 17, 1862. The rest of the war, Company K served with the 50th.[20]

The Confederate Regimental Histories Directory listed John, along with his brothers Doctor Floyd [Doctor Floyd was not a medical doctor, but was given that name, which was widely used in the mountain region during that time.], Elijah, Ephraim, Reed, and Robert, as well as Orlean's brother William, in the 50th Virginia Infantry, Company K, under the command of Captain Jefferson Thompson Lawson.

Andrew Hawks, another of Orlean's brothers, was recorded in the Directory's Muster Roll of the 152nd Virginia Militia.

May Belle T. Smith wrote, "The John Puckett who married Orlean Hawks was in Company K, 50th Virginia, according to his widow's pension application."[21]

On page 319 of the Carroll County Law Order Book for the period September 18, 1911-September 22, 1914 this March 12, 1914 entry was made:

"The following is a list of pension applications examined and approved and ordered to be certified to the Auditor Public Account."

Orlena [Orlean] Puckett's name was on the list. Her residence was given as Gladesboro, Virginia. However, Orlean did not live in that neighboring community. Since, in 1914, the Gladesboro Post Office was probably the closest post office to Orlean's Hillsville home, it is understandable that her address would have been given as Gladesboro.

Smith noted that John's brother Reed joined Company K on June 22, 1861 at Wytheville, Virginia and was "sent to White Sulphur Springs, sick, September 12, 1861. Prisoner of war at Strasburg September 23, 1864. Arrived at Harpers Ferry, Virginia, October 3, 1864, exchanged March 17, 1865. Paroled at Point Lookout, Maryland and transferred to Aikens Landing, Virginia March 17, 1865 for exchange."[22]

Reed, according to David Puckett, "was wounded in the Civil War. He couldn't use his right arm because of a bullet wound."

Doctor Floyd, Smith wrote, joined Company K on June 22, 1861 at Wytheville and "left Wytheville sick August 12, 1861 for [a] 12 month period."[23]

David Puckett explained that Doctor Floyd's death was caused by "Black Irish Syphillis, a bacterial infection not related to a sexually transmitted disease, but a result of a gunshot wound that became infected."[24]

Relatives have been unable to locate Doctor Floyd's grave. However, many believe that he is buried at Hollywood Cemetery in Richmond, Virginia. A letter from the Hollywood Cemetery Company dated August 18, 1998 states:

> *We have searched our files and have found no record of his having been buried in our cemetery. The possibility remains, however, that he was buried in Hollywood, for we only have record of about 7,000 of the 18,000 Civil War soldiers buried here. If he was killed in 1864, his records may be among the ones that were lost in the fire after the Civil War. We lost a total of 11,000 names of soldiers in the fire.[25]*

Doctor Floyd, John's older brother, married Elizabeth "Betty" White on July 17, 1854. By 1860 the couple had five children. The youngest, a girl named Sarah, died on November 10, 1860 at the age of four months. Martha, who was born in 1859, died of diphtheria. She was around a year old.

"Doctor Floyd and Aunt Betty lived in a cabin at the Bent, located close to Meadows of Dan," said David Puckett.[26]

Daughter Elizabeth Matilda "Tilda" was born on August 20, 1861, two months after Doctor Floyd's enrollment in the infantry. He never lived to see Tilda.

Smith indicated that John's brothers Elijah, Ephraim, and Robert also joined Company K on June 22, 1861 at Wytheville, Virginia. Smith recorded the following military entry about Robert:

> *Serve[d] one year. He was born in Carroll County, 36 years, 6 feet 1 inch, light complexion, blue eyes, red hair, a farmer. During the last two months has not been fit for duty. Afflicted with chronic hepatitis for several years, has been gradually growing worse since he entered service — discharged June 25, 1862 at Rocky Gap, Virginia.*[27]

Confederate Pension Rolls of Veterans and Widows listed John's brother Ephraim as disabled. His pension application date was 1902.

Two brothers served in other units. Riley was a private in Company E and Hosea was in Company I. John had five more brothers, but no military information on them is available. Churchill and Jubal died in 1862. Churchill was 29 years old at his death, but Jubal was only 12. Lewis died in 1863 at the age of 36. Another brother, Jacob, was born in 1848 and died in 1920. It is conceivable that Churchill, Lewis, and Jacob could have been in the Civil War. The remaining brother, George Washington, died before the Civil War.[28]

Apparently John's time in the army was short. After the romance and intrigue of war faded, he, like many others, became a deserter. To the deserters, North Carolina Governor Zebulon Vance's sentiment that the conflict was "a rich man's war and a poor man's fight" must have rung all too true. Added to that belief were several other things that made army life unbearable for the soldiers and caused them to desert.

> *The Southern soldiers' main course was cornbread, fried in a pan, and salt beef ('salt horse' as the soldiers called it). The meat was of poor quality and had to be soaked or boiled to remove the salt before it could be eaten. Poor rations led to disease and desertion.*[29]

Unsanitary living conditions and lack of medical supplies contributed to diseases such as malaria, measles, dysentery, and pneumonia:

> *The four D's combined to continually reduce the [Rebel] units' strength; (death, disability, disease, and desertion). Before the Northern armies could invade the South, the Southern army was invaded by rats, fleas, ticks, lice, and other insects. Very little was known about sanitation and communicable diseases. Measles, mumps, and dysentery caused the first casualties of the war. Disease would debilitate and kill more Southern soldiers than Union bullets.* [30]

Added to that was the lack of equipment, pay, and clothing. According to the book *Desertion During the Civil War* by Ella Lonn, soldiers often went barefoot, even in the harsh winter months, sometimes wrapping rags or straw around their feet for needed warmth and protection.

> *It was not unusual to require them to march under such conditions fifty miles a day. As a feeble substitute for shoes, the men flocked to the cattle-pens when cattle were being butchered for food, to cut strips for moccasins before the hides were cold. But the moist, fresh skins without soles slipped about so that the wearers, constantly up and down, would*

finally kick them off to wrap their feet in rags or in straw or to limp along barefoot.[31]

The soldiers' pay, according to Lonn, was "a paltry sum of eleven dollars a month in Treasury notes [and] was almost always delayed. A private's pay for a month would scarcely buy one meal for his family or a year's pay buy him a pair of boots."[32]

"Some deserters from the Civil War had signed up in two different regiments of the Confederacy in order to get their muster money. Then, when they deserted, they were deemed deserters by one side," David Puckett commented.[33]

Lonn wrote:

Added to physical want and depression on the part of the soldiers were homesickness and mental anxiety concerning their families, whom they knew to be in need of the necessities of life in the face of ever-soaring prices: flour, fifty dollars a barrel; salt, sixty to seventy cents a pound; bacon, seventy-five cents a pound; and butter, twelve dollars a pound. With the poor mountain whites, the margin of food supplies from a five-acre farm was always necessarily small.[34]

Additionally, worry over home and family was a great concern of the Confederate soldiers. In her book *Behind the Blue and Gray,* Delia Ray wrote:

While many soldiers could tolerate their own difficulties, they could not bear to remain in the army knowing that their families suffered while they were away. Letters from wives and relatives frequently brought bad news of sickness, failing crops, or lack of food and money. Since most of the war was fought on Confederate territory, southern soldiers had more reasons to worry about their families."[35]

A significant event that could have added to John's homesickness and prompted his desertion from the army was the sickness and imminent death of his daughter. On September 27, 1862, little Julia Puckett, John and Orlean's firstborn, died from diphtheria. She was only seven months old.

There has been some speculation as to who attended Orlean when she gave birth to the child. Wavy Worrell mentioned that "Aunt Orlean's mother-in-law, Granny Sally, lived near them in The Hollow. She's probably the one helped deliver Aunt Orlean's babies, but there was a midwife named Granny Jane Hendrick. She chewed tobacco."[36]

Granny Jane, who would have been around 29 years old at the time, lived only a stone's throw from Orlean. True to the midwife stereotype, Granny Jane dressed in black and also smoked a pipe and dipped snuff.

Orlean's great grandniece, Dee Spellings, remembered that her mother told her "Aunt Orlean would take her [baby Julia] and set her out in the cornfield while she worked."[37]

Several people agreed that Aunt Orlean spent a great deal of time hoeing corn for a pound of fat a day. Wavy Worrell explained that Orlean used the lard [fat] she earned "to cook with, make biscuits, grease pans and such. Said she could beat any man in the field."[38]

Those are almost the same words Reverend C. C. Haymore used when he recounted a conversation with Orlean for *The Republican* newspaper in 1900: "She makes a regular hand in the field and said no man could go ahead of her."[39]

Wavy laughed and told of a time when Orlean was hoeing corn and looked up and saw the moon. "She said it was the first time she'd ever seen the moon in the daytime."[40]

Julia's first symptom of diphtheria probably would have been a low-grade fever. Other symptoms of the disease include rapid pulse, enlarged neck glands and, occasionally, a thick, yellow discharge from the nose. However, the most characteristic symptom is a grayish membrane on the throat and tonsils that can be very dangerous. If the membrane becomes large enough, it can cause croup or, as it most likely did in Julia's case, even prevent breathing. In that pre-vaccine era, there would not have been an antitoxin or antibiotics to treat diphtheria, which was one of the most common causes of death among children.[41]

John was at home when Julia developed the disease. Icy Vass, great grandniece of John and Orlean and sister of Foy Hawks, said that John was grief stricken. He held the infant in his arms and paced the floor all night long before she died.[42]

It is understandable that, after such a tragedy, John would not have wanted to leave Orlean and return to the war. He was just one of many Virginia men who fled the war. House Executive Documents ranked Virginia third in its high count of officers who deserted during the Civil War. The total number of Virginia males that deserted is given as 12,071, with officer desertion totals being 84.

Lonn wrote of the war deserters' hideouts:

> *Shelter was sought, naturally, in remote places, difficult of access, where escape was easy and pursuit difficult: in the gorges and cliffs of mountain retreats...in caves hollowed out from a low hillside or even under the level soil.*[43]

"A whole lot of them [mountain men] deserted and hid out," explained Wavy Worrell. "John would hide out in a cave in the mountains called Salt Peter Rock. He was a war deserter, and Aunt Orlean would take him and the others something to eat. She always whistled to let them know she was coming."[44]

According to David Puckett, one time when Orlean was taking food to John, the Home Guard caught up with her. Later, she told her family that she had been so frightened that it scared the whistle right out of her.

David revealed that there are two graves at Salt Peter Rock, and speculated that they might be those of some Home Guard.[45] While this has not been proven, given the reputation of the Home Guard and their mistreatment of the mountain people, it is possible.

"Home Guard, Pinkertons, Patrollers, they were all the same," exclaimed Marvin Hawks. "They used to take food."[46]

"Detail Troops [Home Guard] came around searching for deserters and stopped at Aunt Orlean's for food," added Foy Hawks. "Aunt Orlean was always generous, but she had to hide food from the soldiers so that she would have some [for herself]. She took food into the hills where deserters were hiding."[47]

"When she'd get groceries [in her later years], she'd put a little bit in one place and some somewhere else," said Wavy Worrell. "She'd hide sugar here and there, around at different places. But we got to thinkin' about it and that was because of the war."[48]

"Well it was on account of the war, you know, when the war was goin' on," retorted Iduna Quesinberry, Wavy's mother. "They expected to be robbed."[49]

Ninevah Willis mentioned this about the Home Guard:

The Home Guard was made up of Southerners who were disabled or too young or old to be in the army. They were also known as Patrollers and Details. They looked for deserters. They mistreated people. Killed animals and robbed people. People would hide food and valuables from them. One family put their valuables in a fruit jar and hid it under a cliff. The Home Guard found it. In it there was a baby's mug, which they broke. The baby cried and cried over that mug. Today the place where the fruit jar was found is referred to as Jar Gap.[50]

On April 9, 1865, the war ended, putting the Home Guard out of business. On that Palm Sunday General Robert E. Lee rode into Appomattox Court House under a white flag and surrendered to General Ulysses S. Grant. In May, remaining Confederate forces surrendered.

The nation was reunited as the Civil War came to an end. Over 620,000 Americans lay dead, with disease having killed twice as many as those lost in battle. Fifty thousand survivors returned home as amputees.[51]

John and his fellow mountaineers were finally freed from worries of war and the Home Guard marauders. They could return to their homes and families and try to resume their former way of life. After the war ended, John abandoned his mountain hideout and reunited with Orlean in their little cabin in The Hollow.

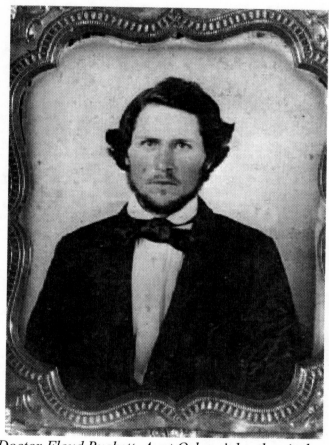

Doctor Floyd Puckett, Aunt Orlean's brother-in-law, who died from wounds received while serving in the Civil War

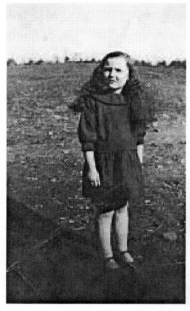

*Aunt Orlean's
great grand-niece
Wavy Worrell*

*Aunt Orlean's
great-niece
Iduna*

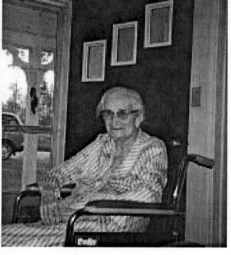

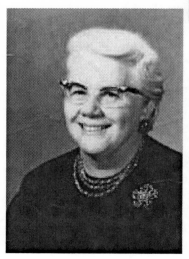

*Neighbor Ninevah J.
Willis, author of Country
Living and Carroll
County educator*

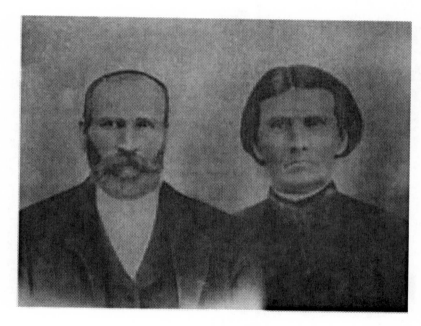

John and Orlean
photo provided by Shelby Puckett

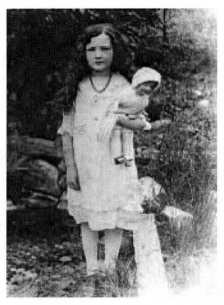

above and right:
Great grand-niece
Wavy Worrell

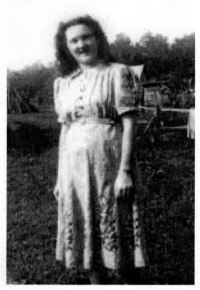

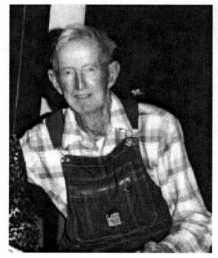

Raymond Pruitt,
neighbor

Chapter 3
The Babies

"I would have been glad if it had been the Lord's will to let one of my children live."—*Orlean Hawks Puckett*

Resettled in their lean-to at the foot of Groundhog Mountain, John and Orlean could once again enjoy nature's bounty and beauty. Those who had traveled afar and returned never would have known that internal changes had taken place in the hills. The mysterious splendor and drunken beauty of the Blue Ridge was as prevalent as ever.

Sallets of poke and cress, beans, onions, and potatoes would have been plentiful, as they are today, in the mountains in springtime. Wild strawberries and huckleberries, there for the taking, were most likely made into pies and eaten after cooling on the kitchen windowsill. Jellies, produced from the berries, sustained families through long winter months, as did Winesap and Horse apples that were dried and stored in pokes and later fashioned into fried, moon-shaped pies or chunky sauces.

With spring came an explosion of color. Flame Azaleas in clusters of orange, yellow, and cream; delicate pink and white blooms of Mountain Laurel; yellow and pink Ladyslippers scattered among the pines; forests of Dogwood and Redbud covered in white blankets of flowering Trilliums; and fields of purple Larkspur and Dwarf Crested Iris, white Bloodroot, and Solomon's Seal, all amid a backdrop of hazy blue mountains and rolling fields, showed the gentle, delicate side of a land that in winter could turn rough and harsh.

Among tangles of laurel and ivy, mountain men hid their stills from the prying eyes of revenuers. Those hardy English and Scotch-Irish descendants could relax with a draught of corn whiskey after a day of hunting wild turkey and deer or fishing in clear mountain streams.

A body could have a good, satisfying life in the hills, free from city folk who didn't know the first thing about planting by the signs or gathering wild greens and herbs. Most flatlanders were unacquainted with the catamount's eerie cry on a long summer night or the touching trek of the wild turkey leading her young to drink from a cool mountain stream. Most likely they'd never experienced the beauty of a mountain sunset when flaming yellow-orange merges with the muted, bluish gray of Appalachia.

Dog days of summer brought in chattering squirrels and chipmunks, whistle pigs, and slow-moving opossums. Wild roses perfumed the thin mountain air and mingled with the fresh scent of balsam and fir. Mounds of feathery wild fern laced the water's edge and carpeted the clean forest floor. The purple-flowering raspberry put forth its red tart fruit. Butterflies and bees flocked to pale purple clusters of Joe-Pye weed and lemon-scented St. John's Wort.

In cabin yards, chickens clucked softly and scratched the dust for bugs. Some mountain men, like John Puckett, worked outdoors among the chickens, using a shaving horse, foot-powered lathe, and joiner to fashion poplar wood into dough boards, rolling pins, buckets, and barrels.

As summer turned to autumn, wood gettin's brought the community together to frolic, feast, and gossip while preparing for the coming, unforgiving winter weather. Chopping wood was always hard work, but the load was lifted when neighbors joined together to complete the chore. Like corn huskin's, wood gettin's were festive occasions complete with food, cider, games, music, and dancing. With all that teamwork, enough wood to last a family through the winter could be chopped and split in one afternoon.

When winter covered autumn's brilliant landscape with drifts of virgin snow, the smell of acrid smoke permeated the land as it curled forth from chinked chimneys. Inside their cozy cabins, mountain families snuggled down among bedticks made of straw or goose feather. Long winter evenings were spent whittling and knitting in front of fireplaces where chestnuts roasted and coffee brewed.

Two winters after the war's end, Orlean became pregnant for a second time. As fall's orange sassafras, yellow hickory, red sourwood, and maroon-colored oaks accentuated by evergreens of pine, hemlock, spruce and fir dotted the mountain landscape alongside rows of ripened cabbages, John and Orlean's baby was born. The child, an unnamed male, was pronounced dead at birth.

In 1868, almost a year later, another son was born to Orlean. Like the last, this unnamed child was also stillborn. Two years passed. Orlean delivered another little girl on October 8, 1870. Sadly, the baby was stillborn. On January 17, 1871 Orlean suffered yet another loss. The child was female. Five months later she gave premature birth to a daughter who survived two days. A child, born four years later, died on April 24, 1875.

Those births were the only ones recorded between 1867 and 1875. However, during a span of 13 years, Orlean Puckett endured 19 pregnancies. It is believed that the unrecorded births were miscarriages. Mrs. Raymond Pruitt, a neighbor of Orlean's who lived along the Blue Ridge Parkway, recalled a conversation she had with Orlean about the babies:

> Now, all of her children was, they was done born 'fore I ever met her. She talked about 'em an' she told me that some of 'em she didn't carry over five months. So, I asked her about the ages of 'em an' she said some of 'em they was just [a few] months difference in the births. They's all close together an' then the two little girls that lived a little while was all that lived of the bunch. I think she told me the oldest, the one that lived the longest was 'bout seven months. I think the other one was [four or five months old]. Those that didn't live was not born natural. Something wrong somewhere. It probably could've been corrected now.[1]

Charlie Bowman, another of Orlean's Parkway neighbors who was interviewed in 1976, concurred with Mrs. Pruitt's recollection of the babies:

I did hear her [Orlean] say that all her children died at birth, you might say. I believe they wuz one that lived just a little bit. I heered them say they was one child lived, but how old she wuz I don't know.[2]

It is understandable that the babies were on Orlean's mind. But, rather than internalize her feelings, she talked openly to friends and family about her grief.

"Seemed like she was worried that she didn't have any [of her own children] that lived," observed Mrs. Dewey Culler, a neighbor who lived near Parkway Milepost 187.5.[3]

Another neighbor, Mrs. Ellis Bowman, reminisced that Aunt Orlean "would talk about her children a heap much of the time. She didn't have any to live, I don't think, but just really three or four months, somethin' like that."[4]

Orlean's great grandniece Hattie Puckett said that the oldest of the 24 children lived to be nine months and that "the rest were born before their time. I think some of them were born dead."[5]

The 19 pregnancies took place during the time that John and Orlean lived in The Hollow. According to Wavy Worrell, the babies were buried at "The Run" in a private graveyard near John and Orlean's lean-to cabin. "That's the Reed Puckett Cemetery," Wavy pointed out, "but Dunkley Puckett owns the land now."[6]

In a 1976 interview, neighbor Charlie Bowman described the cemetery:

I've seen where she's [Orlean] buried, and I have been down at the Doe Run Church [in The Hollow] and seen where her children are buried. I went there this year. It is the first time I have been down there. There's two markers. There's a big long row of graves and there's one marker on each end. And one marker says, "John, born 1882" and "Julia

Ann, born 1861." Somebody said that she put up a marker for the one that was born first and one that was born last. [There is some question as to the accuracy of the inscription "John, born 1882."] All the others just have rocks. Back in them days and times they wuzn't a whole lot of markers put out. Just like in the cemetery right up here in the field. They's been rocks there, but they hasn't been no markers put up to any of the monuments.[7]

In 1875 John and Orlean moved from their lean-to cabin in Patrick County to the top of Carroll County's Groundhog Mountain. One year later another child was born, but died the following day. Four more births were recorded: A live birth that resulted in death on April 10, 1877; a live birth that resulted in death in January 1878; a female child that lived one day and died in June 1878; and a male child that was stillborn in October 1881.

Of those five babies, one was buried with the 19 others in Reed Puckett Cemetery. The remaining four were buried on top of the mountain in Jake Puckett Cemetery, a private graveyard.

The "Report of Preservation of Mountain Culture, Marking of Historic Sites and Promotion of Handicraft, Blue Ridge Parkway" states that "She [Aunt Orlean] gave birth to 24 children. Ten of them were stillborn and all the others died under seven months of age."

The babies' deaths were a mystery to the mountain folk who, whenever Aunt Orlean gave birth, were heard to say, "You better go see Aunt Orlean's baby now if you want to see it a-livin'."

There were cruel rumors, born out of fear and ignorance, that Orlean killed her babies by smashing their heads against rocks. Others said that her hard-drinking husband beat her when she was pregnant and that was why none of the children lived.

Those who knew and loved Orlean didn't believe any of those rumors. They were inclined to think the tragedies were a result of an underlying medical condition. Hattie Puckett declared that Orlean "had some kind of liver trouble or somethin' like that that caused it [the death of the babies]. Her niece had the same problem. She had seven children that never lived."[8]

It was Orlean's dream to have children. In Reverend C. C. Haymore's letter to The Republican newspaper he wrote:

> *In conversation with Mrs. Puckett, she told me that she was 55 years old and had buried 24 children; had just come from the foot of the mountain where she had been to visit a graveyard where 20 of them were buried. She modestly said that she would have been glad if it had been the Lord's will to have let one of her children live.*[9]

Friends and family often heard Orlean say, "I wish the bird [stork] would fly by my door," and Hattie Puckett commented that "Aunt Orlean loved children. Helped family members take care of children."[10]

In those years, when medical knowledge was limited, it must have been hard to fathom why none of Orlean's babies lived. Now medical research has shed a light on what most probably was the source of Orlean and John Puckett's sorrow. According to medical experts, blood typing did not come into existence until the late 1800s. Before then, one would not have known if they were Rh-negative or Rh-positive. The combination of an Rh-negative mother and an Rh-positive father could result in stillbirths, miscarriages, pre-term dead babies, and low pH babies with poor lung development caused by fluid in the chest. It is most likely that Orlean was Rh-negative and John Rh-positive.

If an Rh-negative mother gives birth to an Rh-positive baby, her immune system may develop antibodies to the Rh factor in her baby's blood. The mother's first child is rarely affected; however, her antibodies will attack the blood system of a second Rh-positive child, causing complications such as anemia, jaundice, brain damage, or death.

Since the antibody formation does not occur until the first few days after birth, Orlean's first child would have lived. Unfortunately Julia Ann contracted diphtheria and died at seven months of age. Because of the antibodies Orlean's body may have developed, any subsequent pregnancies would have resulted in newborns with the deadly Rh hemolytic disease.

According to Wayne Rossi of Sera-Tec Biologicals, Rh hemolytic disease usually takes one of three forms. With congenital hydrops, or severe anemia and swelling, the result is usually stillbirth or death within a few hours of birth. Severe jaundice, also called icterus gravis, has a 75 percent fatality rate without treatment. The third form, congenital anemia, is the least serious and can now be treated successfully with Rh-negative blood transfusions. Of course, in Orlean's time there would not have been a treatment for Rh hemolytic disease.

Since the introduction of Rh Immune Globulin in 1968, the buildup of antibodies in the mother can be prevented. Rossi reports that standard medical practice now requires Rh Immune Globulin as a part of prenatal care for all Rh-negative mothers. An immunization is given at 26 weeks gestation and again at post partum. When treated properly, an estimated 95 to 99 percent of all Rh incompatibility and resulting Rh hemolytic disease of the newborn can now be prevented.[11]

Great-great grandniece Shelby Inscore Puckett voiced the belief, shared by many, that there was indeed a medical explanation for the death of Orlean and John's children:

> *For many years numerous explanations have been given for the fate of Aunt Orlena's [Orlean's] 24 babies. One of the most plausible explanations is that of an incompatible Rh blood factor. Medical sources indicate that if the mother has a negative Rh factor and the father is Rh positive, the first child of such a union does not encounter problems. However, subsequent children are in real danger. The birth and death pattern of Orlena and John Puckett's children fit the medical model of incompatible Rh factor since the first child of Orlena*

and John did live for several months before dying of a then common disease while none of the other babies lived beyond birth.

Whatever the cause of death, a row of 20 unmarked field stones in an abandoned family cemetery stands as a reminder of the heartache suffered by this woman. But the Puckett Cabin stands as a very public monument to 'Aunt' Orlena Hawks Puckett's strength and determination as she overcame her own adversity and devoted her life to helping other women achieve what she could not.[12]

Chapter 4
John and Orlean

"First month honey. . .Next month pie. . .
Third month. . . 'Get out here and work, you damn bitch, same as I'."
Orlean Hawks Puckett

Over the years John and Orlean's relationship was sometimes volatile. Orlean often spoke to neighbors and family members about arguments the two had that were usually followed by reconciliation. Some neighbors recalled conversations in which Orlean said that John physically abused her. Orlean once confided in her neighbor, Mrs. Ellis Bowman, about problems she had with John:

> *She would talk a heap about her husband, about the way he treated her and the places he'd go. He wouldn't go to the store and get things. . . coffee, sugar . .that she had to have, so she would get bothered and she would say well, if he couldn't go to the store she could. She would get up on a horse and take her eggs and here she would go get her groceries. I don't know how she ever made it if she was kicked out and treated like she said she was, but I reckon it's because she was strong, you know, stout, and she had a strong ambition and, at the same time, I reckon she had a strong responsibility.[1]*

John did, according to a story told by Wavy Worrell, make a few trips to the store:

> *John got to goin' takin' her butter and eggs to the store to buy groceries and he'd give some of 'em [the butter and eggs] to another woman. Aunt Orlean said that she never cussed but one time, but*

she said, "I'd be damned if I won't do my trading myself [from now on]".[2]

That didn't stop John from going to the store. Coy Martin remembered that, in later years, John "had a cane he walked with, you know, an' he wore a great long beard. He was too old to work when I knew him, but he was still able to walk from out there to my Dad's little ole country store."[3]

Neighbor Raymond Pruitt did not recall any conversations with Orlean about John's mistreatment of her. "I knew him," Pruitt said in a 1976 interview. "He farmed the land, jus' like people did back them days. He had several acres in there. I went a bee huntin' with him one time an' I remember that mighty well. Cut the bee tree. I'm not goin' tell the tale about that one."[4]

In the early years of their marriage, John and Orlean often traveled by train to Bedford, Virginia to visit her relatives. According to Wavy Worrell, John and Orlean's brothers would get drunk during those visits:

One time she took a notion to come home. Well, she kept some money pinned up in her pocket to have a way to get back home when that happened. And John said, 'Yeah, how you goin' get back? You ain't got no way [no money].' And she said they'd be a way.

When she'd get mad at John she'd leave him and go to her family [when they were still living a short distance away in Lambsburg]. John would have Granny Puckett [Betty] go talk to her and beg her to come home. Aunt Orlean would have a shirt made for him as a make-up gift to take back with her.

John went to Big Island, Virginia and worked for a few months. Don't know what kind of work he did there. He used to make dough trays

*and sell 'em. He made the split white oak baskets
that Aunt Orlean carried her eggs in. She traded at
Marshall, Kinzer, Martin, Noonkesters, and Keno
stores and there was one atop Fancy Gap. Keno
and the one atop Fancy Gap is still there.*[5]

Malicious rumors about the deaths of John and Orlean's babies
continued to spread over the years. One neighbor, who shall remain
unnamed, said of the children: "I don't know what was wrong with
them, but some said that they was cruelly mistreated. All along, before
her children were born, her husband, I think, was a little bit on the heavy
side of drinkin'."

Another anonymous neighbor revealed in a 1976 interview that
she didn't know John, but she had heard gossip about John's abusive
nature. "She said that she didn't think he treated her a bit right. He was
mean to her. I don't know. That's what she told this colored woman
down here. I don't know if it was real or not. I never knowed of her
tellin' stories."

"One time when Aunt Orlean had a miscarriage, he [John] locked
her in the house and someone came by and found her and gave her
water and something to drink," remarked another neighbor, who shall
also remain unidentified. "She said that they would fuss and fight when
John drank."

A relative laughed and said that she had heard over the years
that "John was good to Orlean and never did beat her, only when he got
drunk." Like Orlean's neighbor, this relative also heard that John locked
Orlean in the house whenever she was sick. She said, "I don't know
why he'd lock her in the house." Orlean couldn't let anyone in because
she couldn't unlock the door from the inside. Her niece devised a way
to take Orlean food and water by crawling underneath the house and
lifting up floor planks.

Coy Martin of Fancy Gap expressed his opinion of accusations
that John was a wife beater in a 1976 interview:

> *I can recollect him [John] pretty well. I heard one time before, she [Aunt Orlean] mentioned it that the ole man John'd whup her once in a while, but I never knowed that to be true. I wouldn't vouch for it, I jus' don't think it's so, but it could have been. He was good to her when I knowed both of 'em together, but after they got home I don't know how much they did.*[6]

Young girls often came to Orlean for advice on wedded life. She had a saying for them that most likely summed up her own marriage:

> *First month honey...next month pie...third month....Get out here and work, you damn bitch, same as I.*

In his book *The Man Who Moved a Mountain*, Richard C. Davids recounted a conversation Orlean supposedly had with Bob Childress' soon-to-be wife, Lelia:

> *Next day, when Lelia told Aunt Orlean she was going to get married, the old granny-woman tried to discourage her. "He's a good man, child," she said finally, "but you've got plenty of time to get married." Lelia knew she [Aunt Orlean] was thinking of her own marriage, of how her man got drunk and beat her, and of her own babies. As magnificently as she cared for others, she couldn't keep her own children alive.*[7]

When some of John and Orlean's relatives and neighbors read Davids' book, they were outraged that John had been depicted as a drunkard and a wife beater.

Great-great grandnephew David Puckett, who often heard his aunts Hattie and Libby Puckett recall memories of their Aunt Orlean, did not believe the accusations:

I find [the beatings] extremely hard to believe. I seriously doubt that he [John] persecuted Orlean. The things she did, going to birthings and sometimes staying for days, and he didn't question her. He didn't seem to be a control freak.[8]

In defense of John, Larma Puckett commented:

I never heard her say that John beat her, but she'd get mad and leave. She would talk about leaving. She'd get mad and make up by bringing him a shirt. John drank, and that might have been when she'd leave. But, I never heard that he was a heavy drinker. Most men did drink back then. Moonshine was made here.[9]

Great grandnephew Foy Hawks pondered over the serious accusations that were made against Orlean and John. "All sorts of tales came out about Aunt Orlean's 24 children. Some said she used a darning needle to kill them. Others said her husband beat her when he was drunk. Of course, none of those tales were true."[10]

Marvin Hawks, another great grandnephew who, during his childhood, lived with Aunt Orlean, agreed:

You know the rumor got out that Aunt Orlean killed all of her kids. My sister Dee said that our Mama told her that every time that Aunt Orlean would lose a baby that you could hear John Puckett cry from mountain to mountain. He would go up on Aunt Orlean's Knob and you could hear him holler and cry from mountain to mountain. He had a loud voice. He would stay up there and holler, moan, and cry. He wanted kids, just like Aunt Orlean did. I don't believe that John beat Aunt Orlean. I don't think that he'd get drunk. Mama looked after Aunt Orlean during her last days. If she had been abused, she'd have told Mama. They probably had their differences, but I don't think he would have beat her. I don't think she would have lived with him if he had.[11]

It does seem uncharacteristic that a strong and independent woman like Orlean would remain with a man who physically abused her or her unborn babies. Whatever differences the two may have had, after John died Orlean was inconsolable. Those who watched her grieve reflected that she was heartbroken over John's death and believed there was no doubt of how much she loved him. Wavy Worrell added, "When he died Aunt Orlean cried so hard and loud that the neighbors could hear."[12]

One neighbor discounted Orlean's grief by declaring that when John died Orlean said, "He always enjoyed a good fire and I hope he's enjoying one now."

It has been said that no one really knows what passes between a husband and wife behind the closed doors of their home. The same can be said of John and Orlean's relationship. However, there were outward signs that John loved Orlean. In 1875, after she had suffered through 19 ill-fated pregnancies, John showed his love for her by building a lovely new home high atop Groundhog Mountain. It was undoubtedly their hope that the move would bring the happiness that had eluded them for so long.

Chapter 5
Groundhog Mountain

"Hard times, hard times, come again no more,
Many days you have lingered around my cabin door,
Oh, hard times, come again no more."
—*Old Negro spiritual composed by Stephen Foster*

John had purchased 155 acres of land on Strawberry Ridge, now known as Groundhog Mountain, from the Bowman family in 1875 prior to Orlean's last five pregnancies. The land possessed a rich bounty of wild strawberries. Fat, grizzly-haired groundhogs, also called whistle pigs because of their loud, sharp cry, roamed the mountain, gorging on wild greens and garden vegetables. Traditionally, the whistle pigs retreat to their burrows in October and don't reappear until February to let mountaineers know how much longer winter will last.

A well-traveled dirt road ran through the Puckett's land. John decided to build their home by that road facing south, about 300 yards from Cherry Tree Ridge where his deceased brother's wife, Betty, and her children had moved.

Wavy Worrell spent many childhood days with Orlean Puckett and had vivid memories of her home:

> I remember Aunt Orlean's house. John built their house on the mountain. It was made of log and sealed with chestnut lumber. It was two-story with two rooms downstairs and two upstairs. I was never upstairs, but mommy told me that logs divided the upstairs rooms and you had to step across the logs to get from one room to the other like that. The ceiling and walls were smoked till they were brown. There was a door at the top of the stairs and she had a flour barrel up there. Flour came in 25-pound bags.[1]

It was quite a journey that Orlean made from her house on the mountain to a store in The Hollow below to fetch the flour that went into that barrel. In Reverend C. C. Haymore's letter written in 1900 to *The Republican* newspaper, he wrote this of Orlean:

> She carried on her hip up the mountain a 25-pound sack of flour and helped fix dinner for me. How different this is from the girls that grow up these days! A remarkable woman indeed.[2]

In the article that included Haymore's letter, a reporter added:

> It [Haymore's letter] refers to a remarkable woman, like we have always imagined the wives of the pioneer settlers to have been, hale, hearty, and with physical powers which fitted them for duties which a pioneer life made incumbent upon them. The women of today, generally speaking, are but dolls in comparison and such women as Mrs. Puckett, are exceptional and difficult to find. Is it true that we are growing wiser and weaker with each generation? Such, it would seem, is the trend of humanity.[3]

Orlean Puckett proved that she was, indeed, a strong woman. Over a span of 20 years she gave birth to and buried 24 babies. At 37 years of age she was probably too worn out to try to conceive again. According to Wavy Worrell, Orlean said that her "womb had dropped."[4] A prolapsed womb would have resulted in feelings of heaviness, occasional backache, and other female discomforts. Such a condition would have made conception less likely, but not impossible.

During that time, most women suffered quietly over their "female problems." Often herbs, such as ginger, chamomile, and red raspberry were made into teas to relieve aches and pains. Wine of Cardui, sold by mail and in some stores, was used for disorders of the womanly organs. The product was described as a "non-mineral, non-intoxicating medicine for sick, weak ladies, with sick female organs." It claimed to build up the female system, relieve pain, and help cramps.

If Orlean suffered physically, she never complained. In fact, her general health was good, with the exception of an occasional bout of colic and the aggravation of dry eyes. For her problem dry eyes she, according to neighbor Nannie Bowman, bathed them in milk.[5] While it is not scientifically confirmed, the fat in the milk could have acted as a lubricant, adding moisture to her eyes.

In a 1976 interview Mrs. Ellis Bowman reflected about Orlean's health and said that sometimes she suffered with spells of colic. To get rid of it, she fasted. Mrs. Bowman noted that although Orlean appeared to be "awful poor and skinny," she was "stout and seemed to have good health."[6]

Still, twenty years of pregnancies and miscarriages would not have left Orlean without deep, emotional scars, and she often shared her heartache with friends and family. Nevertheless, the remarkable woman forged onward, working side by side with John as they made their home on Groundhog Mountain.

According to Wavy Worrell, John built the staircase in their home. It "was made of walnut and was straight with a banister and was to the right of the front door," she explained.[7]

Marvin Hawks, Orlean's great grandnephew whose family lived with Orlean until her death, added:

> *The staircase was walnut and was pretty. It had a rail, nice stained walnut. They [his parents and Orlean] used to get after our hides for sliding down that banister.*
>
> *I lost my eye on the stairs of that old house. My mother had springs out of the window shades nailed up to hang her towels and things on and one end had come loose. My brother and I were up there playing and I got a hold of that thing and gave it a pull. I was five years old. The end of it came loose*

and drove right in under the side of my right eye and they said it split the eyeball wide open. Mama said they held me for two weeks and pulled all of the eyelashes out of my eye.

The best I can figure, I must have been somewhere around five years old when we moved from the old cabin [former home of Betty Puckett] to Aunt Orlean's house. We called it the big house. Everette [his brother] would have been nine, 'cause there's four years difference in us. The house faced the Parkway. It had two windows and two doors. The chimney was in the middle. Her house was big. Each room downstairs was around 14 x 14. The house was 35 or 40 feet long.

There was a chopping block in front of the house. She used that to get up on the horse. The outhouse was behind the house. The garden, milking place, chicken house, and cellar house were across the Parkway. The cellar house was dug back in the ground and had a roof. They used rail fences, but most were brush fences to keep the cattle in. Had a rail fence across the road. At one time, Jim Collins [Larma Puckett's father] lived up there in Aunt Orlean's house. He sealed the back room and she gave him a bedspread for doing that. He married Dora Bell Puckett, so he was related [to Aunt Orlean] by marriage.[8]

Wavy Worrell said that Orlean's house was never painted. "The kitchen had a half door to keep the cats out," she explained. "She had cats to kill the mice."[9]

Mrs. Lackie Pruitt said in a 1976 interview that the Orlean kept the bottom half of the door closed to keep the chickens out. The upper door was left open so that air could circulate in the house.[10]

Marvin Hawks disagreed with Mrs. Worrell and Mrs. Pruitt about the kitchen door and said that it had a cat hole in the bottom to accommodate Orlean's three cats. A traumatic experience he had as a child etched the vision of Orlean's kitchen door in his mind:

> *This lady named Beulah Quesenberry, who lived over there [below Orlean's house],would walk down to the mailbox and she always played with us. We thought the world of her. One day I was peeping out of that cat hole, watching for her, and didn't see her and she didn't know I was there. She opened the door and tore my fingernails off. Pushed the door up over my fingers. Boy, she squalled and I squalled.[11]*

Wavy Worrell explained the house in more detail:

> *That door [the kitchen door] and another one faced the road. There were two windows on each side of the doors. After John died more windows were added on. Her cook stove was small, had four eyes. It had four little openings or knobs, a fire door and a stove hearth in front with a door underneath to take soot out. The firebox was up over the oven in front. It was black with a yellow door. On the side it had a picture of Benjamin Franklin on the door, a stone fireplace with a hawk's wing hanging up there to fan the fire with, you know.[12]*

Orlean's fancy stove also held a water tank, which warmed the water. David Puckett pointed out that she was the first woman in the community to have a store-bought cook stove and speculated that was one of the reasons she cooked for so many people. He added that Orlean had a very nice home.[13]

When John built the house, he placed the chimney at one end, but there were problems with it because it wouldn't draw out the smoke.

That was the reason the walls inside were brown. John decided to build a new chimney in the center of the house. The fireplace was made of rock and was open to both main rooms. In those days, people used white mud on rock fireplaces to make them white. The fireplace was the dominant feature in the Puckett home, as it was in all other mountain homes. It served as the main heating and cooking source and was the place most families gathered to socialize. Wavy Worrell described the interior of Orlean's house:

> A clock sat on the mantel. There was a long table in the kitchen covered with an oilcloth with a horn of plenty design. She used a cloth one when company came. There were straight chairs, a bed in the corner, rockers, a wash stand for the water bucket and pan — she washed her hands in a tin wash pan — and a wood box. Had a black iron and a knife box for her knives and forks. She slept in the kitchen. Was some small oil lamps with pewter handles. She never had electricity or a phone. Coy Martin carried lamp oil to her from his father's store.[14]

Martin's store sold a line of homemade drugs such as castor oil and Swamp Root. The swamp root plant was a grass that was made into a tea, bottled and used to treat kidney disorders and sore throats.

Coy Martin said in a July 13, 1976 interview that people in the community depended on the old-fashioned remedies they found at his father's store:

> I've known them to come wake him up at night an' want to get into the store to get a bottle o' medicine. Everybody'd have a bottle o' medicine in the house.

> She [Orlean] bought her lamp oil an' coffee [at my Dad's store]. Sometimes she'd get a little salt an' I recall one time she bought a sack of flour. I

guess that's about the first wheat bread there was in the country. She bought a sack o' flour an' I carried her lamp oil can an' she carried the flour. I went home with her. I was five years old. Sack o' flour, I couldn't carry it. It weighed 25 pounds.

Walk all the way with her out there, called it two mile. Usually, you know, when I got there why when she opened the door I'd hand her the oil can an' I headed back the road home.

I don't recollect too much about it [the house], but I've been in it a lot o' times. She had a latch that when she went in that had a string from the latch through a hole in the door. She could pull that latch an' push the door open an' go in an' then when she got in she'd let that latch back down, you know. An' if she didn't want nobody to get in that night, why she'd pull that string back on the inside an' nobody could reach the string to pull that latch up. Sometimes [when I carried the oil can] she'd put a little molasses on a piece o' bread an' give me somethin' to eat.

She sometimes would come to the store with a chicken under her arm an' a little white oak split basket with a dozen eggs in it an' she'd swap that fer coffee, sugar, an' a little salt an' sech things that she had to have. [My Dad would] coop it [the chicken] up 'til he went to Mount Airy in a wagon. He went about every two weeks. He'd take them chickens to Mt. Airy an' sell 'em. That's the way he got his money back. They'd weigh it an' they'd get two or three cents a pound for it, three or four. Forgot jus' what, not over seven cents a pound. They would trade it out, you know.[15]

47

According to Wavy Worrell, Orlean also purchased green coffee beans from the store, which she parched in an iron skillet over an open fire. After they were parched, the beans were ground in an old-fashioned coffee grinder and used to make a pot of fresh coffee.[16]

Larma Puckett pointed out that Orlean "would boil herself a pot of coffee, stand there at the stove and drink it. She could drink more [coffee] than anyone I ever seen in my life."[17]

The large cans of coffee beans Orlean purchased usually held gift incentives, such as cutlery. Iduna Quesinberry, Orlean's great niece, reminisced about some case knives John and Orlean found among their coffee beans:

> Uncle John was my great uncle. He wuz brother to my grandfather. He had two of 'em [knives] on the table and I picked one up, lookin' at it, and he said, "You can have that knife if you want it." Well, he had another one and [my brother] Coy wanted it and I went back to the house and asked him [John] for that knife for Coy. He hollered out just as big, "Take it on, then!" He had a voice, now I tell you he did!
>
> John used to sit at the back door and talk to himself. I never did know what he was talkin' about. I wadn't much size. I don't know, I wadn't no greater than nine years old, don't reckon.[18]

Just around the kitchen corner from where Orlean ground her coffee beans was a hallway. It was wide enough to accommodate two old-timey pie safes. The pie safes were made of maple wood and had metal doors. They were so tall they almost reached the ceiling. In one safe, Orlean stored her canned goods and jellies. Wavy Worrell mentioned that Orlean made delicious sweet pear preserves, which she kept in crocks, and apple jellies. Once, after Wavy told Orlean how much she liked her apple jelly, she sent her a jar. The other pie safe was where Orlean kept her burial wardrobe.[19]

"She kept them clothes in there ever since I can remember," said Larma Puckett. "She would drag them out and I'd say, 'What are you goin' to do with 'em?' You know how kids will do. She said, 'That's what I want to be buried in' and as far as I know, that's what she was buried in."[20]

The other downstairs room in Orlean's house held a dresser, a highboy, a rope trundle bed, a rope four poster feather bed with a foot ruffle, and a rocking chair. Orlean covered the beds with pretty counterpanes [bedspreads] edged in lace.

Rope beds had frames with holes, spaced nine to ten inches apart, on all sides. To make the frames, the rope was knotted at one end, then threaded through the holes from the top end to the bottom end. Next, the rope continued around the frame and was threaded back and forth, from side to side, until the pattern of woven squares was complete. The end piece was secured in a knot to one of the woven ropes. A straw tick or feather mattress could then be placed on top of the rope frame.

The two upstairs rooms, which were rarely used, completed John and Orlean's splendid home.

By all accounts, Orlean was a hard worker. In fact, she worked so hard that John gave her the nickname "Cupin," which means workhorse. Wavy Worrell remembered a story her mother, Iduna Quesinberry, told her about Orlean's nickname:

> *George Puckett, mommy's uncle, came in from Seattle, Washington where he lived and owned a salmon-canning factory. It was 30 years before he came back to Virginia to visit. He passed by Aunt Orlean's house and saw her standin' in the front door. He said, 'There stands old Cupin,' just where I left her.'*
>
> *She washed her clothes outside in a black wash pot. She never used a washboard, said she made her clothes wash themselves, you know. She*

49

*rubbed them together. She was so clean. She'd
come home and take her clothes off and wash 'em.*[21]

Larma Puckett observed that Orlean was so fastidious that she wouldn't let her clothes "get cool from takin' them off until she had them washed and hung up to dry."[22]

Since she didn't have a clothesline, Orlean draped her clothes across bushes to dry. There were several large bushes that stood close by her house. "There's a picture of Aunt Orlean standing by a blood drop bush and there was a purple laurel bush away from the house called 'Uncle John's laurel bush,'" mused Wavy Worrell. "And a cinnamon vine that had something that looked like potatoes on it."[23] Other bushes included a snowball and a rose.

According to Wavy, John made the wash troughs that were used in their springhouse. "John bored holes in the wood troughs. The holes had stoppers in 'em. Aunt Orlean would wash her butter there."[24] Rinsing the milk from the butter made it taste fresher and helped it to keep longer. Salt was often added to enhance the flavor.

Equipped with the troughs that John made, the springhouse was a convenient place for Orlean to churn butter. It, along with the cellar, was located across the road from John and Orlean's house. There was a deep spring on that side of the road and a branch ran through the springhouse. The cool water helped to maintain the proper temperature for storing dairy products and preserving perishable foods.

After Orlean milked her cow, she strained the milk through a cloth and poured the milk into a crock, covered it and let it stand until the cream rose to the top. After a few days, the cream was skimmed off. When enough cream was gathered, the churning took place. A wooden dasher was used to stir the cream in the churn until it turned into butter.

A chant often accompanied the butter-making ritual: "Come butter, come. Come butter, come. Peter standing at the gate waiting for a butter cake. Come butter come."

After the butter was washed, it was pressed into molds. Any liquid that remained in the churn was buttermilk. Iduna Quesenberry remarked that Orlean "used a long-handled dipper, I think, to dip her buttermilk out. It was a metal dipper."[25] Buttermilk was good to drink or to use when making biscuits. If the skimmed milk soured or "clabbered" it was also used in biscuit making.

In addition to the deep spring that fed the branch through Orlean's springhouse, Marvin Hawks mentioned another spring across the road from Orlean's house:

> *Back in the 30s when a drought hit, people came from all around to the Flat Rock spring to get water. The Parkway put a culvert in and it filled the spring up. At that time the Parkway offered to put a well in for Daddy anywhere he wanted it because they polluted his water. He was good to them and just said put a ditch in to keep it out and we had to move down and start using the other spring.*
>
> *She [Orlean] used a spring across the road. There were three springs over there. What we called a big spring, a middle spring, and a rock spring. Now this little rock spring has water that boils straight up out of it. All three springs are still there.*[26]

The three springs were a life force for the mountain community. Thirsty passersby could reach for the hollowed out gourd that hung on a tree near the big spring and partake of its cool, clear water. According to Iduna, buckets were used to carry water from Flat Rock spring. "She [Aunt Orlean] had two paper buckets," explained Iduna. "Well, like it was wax, you know. One was a yeller lookin' one and one was a sort of red lookin' bucket. I guess it'd hold about three gallons of water."[27]

The springs were a danger to those who couldn't swim. Iduna reminisced that "Dorrie Collins washed down there [at the big spring] one time and she went to pick up a big ole pan full of water and liked to fell in."[28]

"We'd go to the spring and carry water up the hill," recalled Hattie Puckett. "It was a big spring. She'd [Aunt Orlean] always tell us to be careful and not fall in that spring. We were little."[29]

Orlean and John wanted a well on their property, so they could cut down on the frequent trips to the spring. Marvin Hawks said that a 60-foot-deep well was hand dug beside of Orlean's house, but no water was found. "They filled it up," he declared, "and we were always cautioned about walking on that well. It was a little sunk in."

Marvin pointed out some large rocks other than the ones at Flat Rock spring:

> *Salt Peter Rock is where John and the others [deserters] hid out. The Resting Rock is down below that by Doe Run Road. Everything looks very different now. It's grown up.*
>
> *On Aunt Orlean's house side there were 31 acres. The Parkway bought it for around $400.*[30]

According to many of Orlean Puckett's relatives and friends, she and John did not live in the one-room cabin on Blue Ridge Parkway Milepost 189.9 that has been identified as her home. Rather, Orlean's two-story home sat a few yards away from the cabin, which belonged to her sister-in-law, Elizabeth White Puckett.

Long time neighbor Raymond Pruitt verified in a 1976 interview that the small cabin was the home of Elizabeth "Aunt Betty" Puckett. "The little cabin that stands on the Parkway as a memorial to Aunt Orlean was the home of Aunt Betty Puckett, who was married to Doctor Floyd. It's been there ever since I can remember."[31]

One relative said that the cabin, identified by the United States Department of Interior National Park Service as Puckett Cabin, started out as a corncrib. It was originally located on a little knoll called Cherry Tree Ridge, which was below the scenic Parkway. After Doctor Floyd's death, John had the transformed, corncrib cabin moved to its current location so that Betty could be near him and Orlean. Many years later, after Betty's children married and moved from home, her granddaughter lived with her.

David Puckett revealed that prior to the Civil War Betty, Doctor Floyd, and their children made their home at "The Bent," an area close to Meadows of Dan:

> *The Pinnacles of Dan are two mountains where dams were built during the Depression to supply power. The Bent is between those two dams. There is a road called Bent Road. After he [Doc Floyd] died in the Civil War, in 1863 or 1864, Aunt Betty lived in a cabin at Cherry Tree Ridge, which is located east of the Puckett cabin on the other side of the Parkway. It was on the original 155 acres John bought from the Bowmans.*

> *Aunt Betty was jolly and a lot of fun. She, like most of the other women in the family, was scared to death of thunderstorms, so John and Orlean decided to move her beside of them. The cabin on Cherry Tree Ridge was moved to its present location.*

> *When Aunt Betty lived on Cherry Tree Ridge, her two sons, Stewart and George, ages 15 and 16, lived there also. One day Jacob "Little Jake" Puckett, Jr., their uncle, gave both of them a good whipping. They left the country [area], setting off to California or Washington.*

> *They didn't tell Betty they were leaving and she didn't know where they were, if they were alive or dead. They didn't return for visits until after Jake Puckett was dead. They must have done something pretty bad to have run off like that without telling their mother.[32]*

According to Wavy Worrell, the two boys received the whippings because, in the mind of "Little Jake" Puckett, they took too long to fetch the lathe he had sent them after.

George and Stewart had moved in with their grandparents to make things easier on their mother. Their sister Tilda was sent to Hillsville, Virginia to live with a wealthy family when she was only eight years old. She did not return to Groundhog Mountain until 17 years later when she married Eli Hawks. Daughters Martha and Sarah had died before Betty moved into the cabin that stood beside of Orlean and John's home. Her two remaining children, Etta and Robert Lee, who was born on December 5, 1869, five or six years after Doc Floyd's death, lived with her in Puckett Cabin.[33]

There has been much speculation as to who fathered Robert Lee. Some believe John Puckett was the most likely candidate, but one source points to a wealthy man who lived in the community.

At the age of 23, Stewart joined the army in Fort Douglas, Utah, where he was a scout in the Indian War. During that time he fell in love with a beautiful Indian girl. After only a short time together the girl departed, leaving behind a brokenhearted Stewart. Disillusioned by love, Stewart headed to California to pan for gold. After spending time there, he joined the Alaska gold rush frenzy. Far from civilization, with only a dog for companionship, he camped out in the Klondike for a year. Some time later he met a woman named Mattie Glass and the two were married onboard a ship. During their marriage Mattie gave birth to a set of twins, but neither of the children lived. The marriage soon dissolved. After making his fortune in Alaska, Stewart went to work as a railroad conductor. For some unknown reason, word spread throughout Carroll County that Stewart had been killed while working on the railroad. However, according to Marvin Hawks, John Puckett did not believe the rumor that Stewart was dead:

> *Uncle John got up one morning and said, "Stewart is coming home today." Everybody said, "No, he's dead." Uncle John sat outside in a chair and watched up the road. He saw this big man coming up the road and said, "Oh hell, it's Stewart coming!" Uncle Stewart came and he thought his*

mother, Granny Betty, was dead. He had just come in on a visit, but when he found out she was still living, he stayed.

People looked up to him because he was the richest man around.

He bought a car, never could drive, and my Dad did all the driving and looked after him when he went blind. Last car he had was a 1935 Chevrolet. First one was a 1928 Pontiac with a rumble seat.[34]

In 1931 Stewart went blind. Wavy Worrell, who was five years old at the time, remembered the circumstances surrounding his blindness:

He had cataracts and his eyes continued to worsen. He was taken to have surgery, but felt they were going to "put him down." He got scared, wouldn't let them perform the surgery. The cataracts caused him to eventually go blind.

I remember there was a big snow and he gave Libby and Hattie [my cousins] ten cents to go to the spring. He could barely see them as they walked across the field.[35]

On April 1, 1939, Stewart died from pneumonia and heart related problems. He was 83 years old.

Like his brother Stewart, George also panned for gold in both California and Alaska, but, according to Wavy, eventually moved on to Seattle, Washington. There he married a wealthy woman named Sybil and together they had three sons and a daughter. George became the owner of a prosperous salmon-canning factory. He lived out the remainder of his years in Seattle.

Betty Puckett was never alone in her tiny cabin along the Parkway. Her last days were spent with son Stewart by her side. When she was a young girl, granddaughter Etta Hawks moved in with Betty and remained there until her 21st birthday. She was married a year later.

Betty's cabin was sparsely decorated. It contained two beds, a kitchen table, and a pie safe where she kept her dishes.

At one time, the roof extended over the front of the cabin. "I call it a shed," explained Iduna. "There used to be a shed come plumb out over the yard. It come plumb on out from the roof of the [cabin] out over the yard."[36]

One side of the cabin was covered with a rose bush. There was also a snowball bush in the front.

At the age of 90, Betty babysat Larma Puckett, who was only a few months old, so that Larma's parents could plant corn. Shortly after that, on May 24, 1917, Betty died. Larma recalled that she and her parents were living with Orlean. "We [Larma and her siblings] used Aunt Betty's cabin for a playhouse. There was a ladder to get up in the loft. We had us a good time."[37]

Betty's granddaughter Iduna could not remember the ladder leading to the loft. "There was a loft up there, but nobody didn't sleep up there. There wadn't no way of getting' up there only you clumb up over the foot of the bed an' swung up. I never was up in the thing."[38] The ladder was probably installed after Betty's death.

Like Larma, Marvin Hawks also remembered a loft ladder. His parents moved into Betty's empty cabin and he and his brother were born there. "After Coy, that was my brother, and Tavia married, they lived there [in Betty's cabin] a long time," explained Iduna. "[When more children] came along, they had to build 'em another house out there in the edge of the woods. They [later] moved in with Orlean."[39]

Marvin described Betty's cabin:

There was a ladder, two windows, one on the side and one at the front of the loft. [The cabin] had one room with a loft for a storage area. She [Betty] put pine knots in the fireplace to start a fire, called them lighter knobs. The front door was kept open a lot to let the light in.[40]

Iduna, who often spent the night with Granny Betty, said that she used lamps to light her cabin:

> *Now I was gonna stay up there one night with Granny and she was gonna learn me how to bake wheat bread the next mornin' and Uncle Stewart he had to go to work and they waked me up and wanted to know if I wanted to put on bread. [At that time, Stewart had moved back home to live with his mother.] I told Granny no, that Uncle Stewart would be late and that she could put the bread on. I didn't get to bake it.*
>
> *Granny Betty cooked by the fire. Made the prettiest little loaves of bread you ever seen and she was paralyzed in one hand. And she could. . .make the prettiest little cakes of bread I ever seen.*[41]

Neighbor Lackie Pruitt commented in a 1976 interview that he visited with Betty and Stewart many times. He said that he knew she didn't have a stove, because he remembered when she fried some country ham for him. "She pulled them coals right out of the fireplace, put a skillet on there and fried that and that was the best ham that I ever eat. That was good!"[42]

Betty and her sister-in-law Orlean worked closely together, performing "women's work" such as baking, housecleaning, making lye soap, and tending chickens.

Like most mountain women, Orlean had many chores to keep her busy. She made lye soap, which she gave freely or bartered for staples. "Neighbors would furnish the grease," explained Wavy Worrell, "and she'd get the lye and take ashes from the fireplace, put 'em in the lye hopper."[43]

The lye hopper was usually a makeshift affair. Sometimes a wooden barrel or hollow tree trunk served as the hopper. Situated on a slanted board, the hopper was lined with cornshucks or straw. Ashes were placed on top of the liner and water was then poured over the ashes. The lye dripped slowly from an opening or spout in the hopper into a trough or bucket.

When enough dripped lye was gathered, it was mixed with grease in a black wash pot which was placed over an open fire. The grease used in soap making could be hardened animal fat called suet. Mutton, beef, or hog tallow was also used.

The lye and grease mixture was stirred as it boiled. After it thickened and cooled, it was cut into squares. Some people believed that soap hardened better when it was made under a new moon.

Other chores included housecleaning. Wavy explained that Orlean used a "privy broom" made from a bush to sweep the yard.[44] Mountaineers weren't bothered with trimming their lawns, since, with the exception of flowers, shrubs, and trees, the yards were barren. Diligent women swept their yards to make their homes look tidy.

Orlean's house was spotless. She kept her uneven wood floors clean and white by using a scrub broom made from witch hazel. She'd throw down some sand, scrub the floor, then rinse it off.

David Puckett said that he'd been told Orlean Puckett was a meticulous woman, who moved her furniture quite frequently.[45]

Some of Orlean's talents seemed better suited for a man. One of them was tanning bark. Wavy said Orlean used juice from bark for tanning sheep and cow hides.[46] The leather was used to make shoes, boots, belts, and saddlebags.

The bark Orlean used for tanning came from the American chestnut tree. The tree's bark and wood were rich in tannic acid and Orlean, like others who tanned bark, used the tannin extract to process animal hides.

The American chestnut tree was of great importance to the Appalachian community. Its brown nuts, gathered in autumn, stained the hands, but provided buying power for an otherwise penniless family. Sold at market, chestnuts brought from two to five cents a pound.

Wavy recalled that her Uncle Albert gathered chestnuts to barter for clothing. "He was five years old. He picked up enough chestnuts, took 'em to the store to buy him a jeans cloth to make him a pair of britches."[47]

Families rose early in the morning to scour the forests for chestnuts, gathering bushels a day that were loaded onto wagons and carried to large trading centers where they were later resold at a much higher price. Most chestnuts made their way by rail car to big cities like Chicago and New York where they were roasted and sold by street vendors. Most mountain children wore shoes that were paid for with chestnuts. The nuts were also exchanged for books and other school supplies.

According to The American Chestnut Foundation, "the tree's consistently heavy nut crop was the single most important food source for a wide variety of wildlife from bears to birds. Native wildlife from birds to bears, squirrels to deer, depended on the tree's abundant crop of nutritious nuts."[48] Mountaineers let their hogs run free to forage on the sweet, meaty chestnuts and fatten up for slaughter. Squirrel meat, frequently served in a stew or pan-fried, was tastier when the animal had fed on the delicious kernels.

In the mountain area American chestnuts were an integral part of the human diet, whether consumed in an indirect way through the animals or eaten directly. Roasted, the nuts provided a tasty winter treat for the entire family.

Not only did the chestnut tree provide food in the fall, its wide-spreading branches produced fragrant and showy cream-yellow flowers in summer. The spectacular tree provided shelter and shade, its massive trunk measuring "up to five feet in diameter and up to 100 feet tall."[49]

Almost every part of the tree was useful. Granny women like Aunt Orlean boiled the canoe-shaped, toothy-edged chestnut leaves into a broth that they used to treat chest coughs and colds.

In addition, chestnut logs provided a uniform heat source. The straight-grained lumber was "lighter in weight than oak. . .and as rot resistant as redwood." Because it was easy to work with, chestnut wood was used in many building projects and was ideal for sealing mountain homes. Orlean's own home had been sealed with chestnut. Split rail fences, footbridges, telegraph poles, railroad ties, shingles, cradles, and coffins were made from the strong wood, as well as musical instruments and fine furniture. It could be said that the American chestnut tree surrounded mountaineers from cradle to grave.[50]

"When John was livin' they had sheep," explained Wavy. "John and Grandpa Hawks would feed the sheep, but they had lambs in a pen and Grandma Hawks would feed them milk on her finger from a pan."[51]

Across from Aunt Orlean's house was a knob called "Aunt Orlean's Knob" where their sheep grazed along with some that belonged to others. John and Orlean owned 19 head of sheep and a few cows. They had a blue shepherd dog to herd the livestock. Shep had a white ring of fur around his neck and was a beautiful old dog. He was trained to drive the sheep and cows home and separate them from the others. John's command to his faithful dog was, "Go get the cows, Shep," and he'd run over into the mountain field and drive the cows home.

Shep was an intelligent and protective dog. Sadly, he contracted rabies and had to be put to sleep. Wavy lamented that Aunt Orlean's brother got rabies, also. "It didn't have nothing to do with Shep," she said. "He lived in Bedford. Had to tie him in the bed. He begged them to let him die."[52]

The sheep were hand-sheared in springtime, usually after the tenth of May. Professional hand shearers traveled through the mountains during that time of year and were paid to do the work. However, the ever resourceful mountaineers soon learned to shear the sheep themselves and often joined their neighbors for community sheep shearings.

After the greasy wool was washed in hot water with lye soap, it was spread out onto the grass to dry. The dried wool was then sent away to be carded.

After the wool was carded, the spinning took place. Orlean knew how to spin, but didn't own a spinning wheel. Since her niece Elizabeth owned one, she depended on her to perform that task. A bobbin was placed on the spindle, the wheel was turned, and the magical process of spinning took place. When enough bobbins were produced for weaving, the strings were made into skeins for easy dyeing.

Placing a skein of spun wool onto a stick, Orlean dipped it into the hot liquid dye. She used various plants, barks, berries, hulls, seeds, and roots to obtain the desired colors. Walnut hulls and sumac berries produced tan or brown shades. Broom straw yielded yellow. When combined with dye flower and dye leaf or horse sugar, the yellow miraculously turned to orange or red. Indigo dye from the indigofera plant harvested blue tones, while pinks and lavenders were derived from pokeberries. Fragrant pine needles and green oak leaves gave green results. The mountain land offered a vast array of resources for wool dying.

Most ladies on Groundhog Mountain and Doe Run were skilled weavers. Using looms, dyed wool was woven into rugs, coverlets, and counterpanes. Sometimes the yarn was woven into dressmaking material. Iduna Quesenberry commented on a dress that was made for her:

> *My mama wove me a lacy dress. Sort of a green and red. Was just one thread of yarn, you know, that she put in and it was pretty, but they had to put a different collar on to keep it from scratchin' my neck.*

> *Now that peach seed coverlet that she [my mama]wove, it was pink and the cotton was white. Mac [the last baby delivered by Aunt Orlean] had his picture made on that coverlet when he was little.*

> *To weave a coverlet, I believe she said it took six [pedals on a loom]. When she wove blankets with black stripes in 'em I think she said she used*

two little pedals with them. It looks funny though to
see 'em move that old shuttle.[53]

In those days, according to Wavy Worrell, the cotton used in weaving was purchased in hanks and woven on a loom along with the yarn. A domestic cloth, which was unbleached cotton, came from a weaving factory in Mount Airy, North Carolina. This was used to make bed sheets. Striped cotton, which was imported from other states, was used to make bed ticks. The ticks were filled with straw or feathers and placed on rope beds.[54]

Weaving was a valued skill that most mountain women loved. Items produced on the loom could be passed on to future generations and this gave weavers a sense of pride and inspiration. Weaving was often considered more important than formal education. "Well, my grandmother said that they gave her a choice to learn to weave or to go to school," confided Wavy, "and she chose weavin' and evidently she was a good hand at it."[55]

Although Orlean didn't spin or weave, she was an excellent seamstress. She was good with stitches and created her own bed sheets. She hemmed her petticoats and dresses by hand and joined in at quilting bees. Wavy explained that Orlean didn't quilt, but "helped the others tack" the quilts. "She tied and clipped."[56]

Quilting bees gave the women of Groundhog Mountain and Doe Run an opportunity to use their creative skills and to socialize. Unlike weaving, which is a one-person task, several women could work together to make a patchwork quilt. Whenever news got out that a young girl was to be married, women in the community gathered to design and make a quilt for the bride-to-be. If a neighbor suffered the misfortune of a house fire, a quilt was lovingly constructed and offered to them.

Patchwork quilts could be pieced, appliqued, or a combination of both. A variety of patterns such as Wedding Ring, Jacob's Ladder, and Bear Paw were used in quiltmaking. Some quilts reflected unique designs by each woman who worked on them. These were called Friendship quilts. Individual squares were fashioned and embroidered with the artist's name. When enough squares were gathered, they were sewn together to become the quilt top.

When the applique method was incorporated into a quilt, a smaller piece of cloth was laid on top of a larger one and hemmed down. Made from a combination of pieced and appliqued sections, a quilt surpassed the definition of ordinary patchwork.

Quilting was achieved by using a frame, suspended from the ceiling, to hold the material in place. The basic material consisted of a bottom lining; a filling or "bat" made from cotton, wool, felt, or other soft material; and the finished top piece. The first step was to temporarily sew the bottom lining onto the quilt frame. Next, the filling was spread evenly over the lining. The quilt top was then placed over the filling and secured to the bottom lining by basting or pinning. Women gathered in chairs around the quilt frame to attach the patchwork quilt top with delicately skilled stitches. The final step was to remove all basting or pins, take the quilt from the frame, turn the lining up over the quilt top edges, and hem it for a nice, smooth finish.

Young girls often begged to be the first to sleep under a brand new quilt. It was believed that when a maiden slept under a new quilt she would dream of her future husband.

John and Orlean's livestock provided food for their table. Meat from older sheep that were slaughtered was called mutton. Wavy said that Orlean disliked the taste of mutton:

> *They ate mutton. Aunt Orlean said she didn't like mutton, but someone cooked a pot of beef and mutton and she ate it and bragged on it. She didn't know she was eatin' mutton.*
>
> *There was a big old log smokehouse where they kept meat and grain. Pigs were slaughtered and the meat cured in the smokehouse. The smokehouse had a heart-shaped lock on the door.[57]*

When hogs were slaughtered during the warm summer months, the meat was preserved by the method of canning. Fresh pork was also cooked and eaten immediately, before it could spoil. Orlean made backbone pie. She mixed pieces of the cooked hog backbone with biscuit dough to make a dish similar to chicken and dumplings.

Typically, hogs were slaughtered in late November. Cold winter temperatures prevented the meat from spoiling while it cured. Most mountaineers killed hogs when the "signs" were right. Those who practiced that method believed meat fried from a hog slaughtered under a full moon wouldn't shrink when cooked and would render just the right amount of grease or lard.

There were several ways to cure hog meat. After slaughtering, while the meat was still warm, it was taken to the smokehouse, salted liberally with rubbing motions, then set aside on a shelf until the salt was absorbed. It was sometimes salted for a series of three days. Some people added black or red pepper and molasses or brown sugar. The meat would keep up to eight weeks, depending on the temperature.

If meat was needed during the winter months, it had to be washed and soaked over night. Then it was parboiled before cooking.

Meat that remained in the smokehouse throughout the winter had to be treated in springtime. After it was thoroughly washed, it was coated with brown sugar and pepper and placed in a cloth bag to hang in the smokehouse.

After cured, salted meat was washed and allowed to sit at temperatures below 40 degrees for 20 to 25 days, it could be smoked. Hickory, oak, or apple woods were the fuel source used in that process, which took an average of two days. Hams were done when they reached an amber or mahogany color.

In addition to sheep and hogs, Orlean also raised chickens. Some were killed and cooked while others were used for laying. Wavy Worrell mentioned that free running chickens were often a nuisance to Orlean:

She'd raise chickens, you know, young chickens. She had a garden pretty close. And the old hen would get out and scratch in her garden and Aunt Orlean took a rock or something, hit its toes to make 'em sore so it wouldn't scratch her garden.[58]

David Puckett recalled hearing that Orlean tied her chickens to a stake in the yard. This also would have curtailed their scratching in her garden. If any of Orlean's chickens fell sick, she depended on her great grandniece Hattie to nurse them back to health.[59]

Wavy described a cure that was used for Orlean's ailing chickens that had a bad side effect:

> *Somebody told Coy, her great nephew, to put a little lye in the chicken's drinking water to cure whatever they had and one old hen, I reckon it was Aunt Orlean's, must of got too big a dose. It eat a hole in her craw. She'd swallow a grain of corn and it'd fall out.*[60]

Orlean bartered the eggs and sometimes the chickens, chestnuts, butter, shelled corn and dried apples for coffee, salt, flour, sugar, ginger, cloth, shoes, and lamp oil. The chickens usually brought between two to four cents a pound.

She was known to make the most delicious chicken and dumplings and chicken stew around. Neighbors would come to Orlean's house for wood gettin's. After enough wood to last through the winter was cut and stacked, the men sat down and enjoyed one of Orlean's famous chicken dishes.

In addition to the eggs and chickens, Orlean also bartered milk. Neighbors traded buckets of ground wheat, known as "chop," with Orlean for her cow's milk.

Since she and John grew very little wheat, she bartered for wheat flour at the store. The flour came in cloth bags and, after the empty bags were washed, they could be used to make curtains, dish towels, children's dresses, and diapers.

Orlean had a reputation for her culinary skills. She made wheat bread and served it with jelly or gravy. She and John grew an abundance of buckwheat, rye, and oats, which they harvested with a cradle [cutting tool]. They ate lots of buckwheat cakes and cornbread.

Orlean loved to eat cornbread and buttermilk. She crumbled the cornbread into a bowl or cup, poured the cold milk on top, and ate the moist mixture with a spoon.

Wavy remembered that Orlean always fed children when they came to her home:

> She fed 'em bread with butter and molasses. Made molasses sweet cakes — used molasses and honey to sweeten bread and things. She made a dip with buttermilk and sugar and put it over pies. One time I was up at Granny's and she brought a whole big kettle full of sweet potato cobbler down there.[61]

Iduna reminisced, "I can remember eatin' her sweet potater pies an' cakes. Boy, she could cook."[62]

She passed on some of her cooking secrets to great grandnieces Hattie and Libby:

> She learned us to help her cook. We put bread on for her. She made bread in the skillet, the old-timey way by the fireplace. She had flat iron pans where she baked bread in the cook stove.
>
> She cooked beans, taters, cabbage. We helped her peel taters. She had iron cookin' pots she cooked them in and then she had a cook stove. Cooked a whole lot of stuff in the fireplace. Had a pot that hung over the fire and could swing it in and out.[63]

John and Orlean grew navy beans and black beans. Wavy said that after the beans were harvested, the community came together to shell them:

> They had bean hullin's and Orlean would cook the beans for soup. She cooked beans and

66

*taters. She would cook up a pot of beans. She
always tried to feed those who stopped by. Mommy's
brother Kim had been a goin' to stay all night with
her when she was alone, but he didn't go one night.
She left his supper on the table, thinking he might
come, and went on to bed. Somebody went in and
eat it, but Kim didn't go that night. Never did know
who it was.*[64]

David Puckett mentioned that Orlean "always kept a big barrel
of salt and whenever anyone ran out they'd go to her house and help
themselves. Orlean was the nicest woman around."[65]

Hattie Puckett remembered Orlean's generosity, also:

*She was a likeable person and always fed
everybody comin' and goin'. If anyone stopped at
her house, she cooked 'em dinner. Didn't matter
who it was, whether she knew 'em or didn't. She
liked people and everybody liked her.*

*She cooked and canned all the time. Made
preserves. Had the awfullest sight of canned stuff.
She made a garden as long as she was able. Made
sweet taters and beans and stuff. We thought the
world of her.*[66]

Foy Hawks said "If anyone visited Aunt Orlean, they never
went away empty handed. She always gave them something, even if it
was just a piece of cornbread."[67]

Mrs. Ellis Bowman recalled that Orlean made sauerkraut:

*Made kraut 'bout as long as she lived. One
time I was up at Aunt Orlean's and thar was about
five boys thar from one family and they'd all been
in service at the same time. We went up thar and got
to her house and they come in and she got out a
bowl of kraut. Oh, a big bowl! And she put a spoon*

*in thar and they sit down and they everyone eat out
of that bowl of kraut. It nearly killed them. It was
sour, you know, and good. Real delicious. They
just eat that and enjoyed it."*[68]

Larma Puckett remarked that most passersby were drawn to
Orlean's welcoming home:

*Everybody considered Aunt Orlean's house
their own. Her house was on the road, so it was a
convenient stop for travelers. It was a good dirt
road in front of her house, about the same place as
the Parkway runs. She had no privacy.*[69]

Irish peddlers traveled through the mountains, plying their wares.
The majority of them walked on foot, carrying their heavy sack of goods
slung over their shoulder. Wavy Worrell remembered them from her
childhood:

*There were always peddlers. Irish peddlers
came by selling lace, cloth, and Indian herbs. One
herb was a brown powder used as a laxative. Aunt
Orlean would fix them something to eat. Peddlers
gave her lace and cloth for feedin' 'em and lettin'
'em spend the night. She had a white linen tablecloth
she used when company came. She got that from a
peddler.*[70]

The peddlers carried goods that mountaineers were unable to
purchase at the local stores. Iduna Quesenberry described one of those
items:

*One time I's up there and the old peddler
come along. He come a talkin' to hisself and he left
that way. I's a little bit afraid of him. But he had
one of the prettiest silk dresses I thought I ever seen.
It was pink. Well, Lord, if I'd had a hundred dollars
I believe I'da give [it to] him for that dress.*[71]

Not all of the people who passed by Orlean's home were trustworthy. One day an old tramp stopped by her house and asked for a cup of hot water to drink. When Orlean handed him the water, she noticed that his hands were covered with blood. She knew immediately that something was wrong and thought, perhaps, he had killed someone. She and Betty were alone on the mountain. They became so frightened that they went to Betty's daughter's house to spend the night.

Orlean worked in the house and out, too. She and John grew hay for their livestock. Wavy Worrell explained how they harvested their hay. "They didn't bale it, like they do now. They mowed it with mowing belts."[72] After the hay was cut, it was spread out in the field to dry. The dried hay was then gathered, using wooden pitchforks, and arranged into stacks. Haystacks remained in the field, while baled hay was stored in the barn. In addition to hay, livestock was also fed fodder, which was dried corn leaves.

Wintertime brought additional chores for Orlean, such as making hominy. It was a time-consuming process. The initial cooking took at least eight hours. The black wash pot was filled with water, lye, and shelled corn, then placed over a fire. Large, white corn kernels produced the best hominy. After the cooked corn swelled and popped open to reveal tender grains, the washing took place. Orlean transferred the grains to a tin pan and washed them thoroughly in water at the spring until all of the husks and lye were removed. The next step was to cook the grains all night long over an open fire. The fire was checked frequently and water added to the pot throughout the night. The end result was tender, tasty hominy.

Orlean and John's garden included a cabbage patch. Iduna and Wavy laughed and said that Orlean was known to set out cabbage one day and hoe it the next. Iduna also laughed about some childhood shenanigans that took place in Orlean's cabbage patch:

> She had a big ole cabbage patch back of
> Granny's ole house. Big ole leaf cabbage. She'd

grow vegetables, sweet taters an' worked hard. She'd have cabbage, sweet potaters, beans.

They had sheep in that back field. Me and my brother Coy went down to feed the sheep. He would carry me on his back through the briar patches. We'd hunt bird nests. Take eggs and string up for necklaces.

We'd go up that ole deep gulley, crawl up a bank and crawl in the cabbage patch and we'd bite the cabbage heads.

They [John and Orlean] thought the sheep was doin' it. Well, they all got to quarrelin' on the sheep bitin' the cabbage heads and they couldn't find no sheep tracks. They didn't know what had been in the garden. They found out, I reckon, it was us a-bitin' the cabbage heads.[73]

Orlean cooked the cabbage in hog lard. She cooked bear grass, branch lettuce, and other greens in lard, also. Marvin Hawks explained that bear grass grew on Buzzard Rock and branch lettuce was found along the creek bank:

Buzzard Rock is below the knob [Aunt Orlean's Knob]. You could see Aunt Orlean's Knob clearly. It [Buzzard Rock] hangs over. It's a big, old slick rock. Bear grass grew down there and was used in a cooked salad. It was coarse. It still grows there. It's hard to get to and the rock has water and it's slick.

Above it [Buzzard Rock] there's a cellar. On down there's branch lettuce. Tastes like watercress. Cut it up, put grease and salt on it.

It was good. [There was] a stinging weed mixed in with it and when you picked it, it'd sting you to death. It was good. Had to get it at a certain time. . .early spring. It was good.[74]

Iduna said that she and her brother Coy used to hunt for bear grass at Buzzard Rock:

> *I been to the top of [Buzzard Rock], but I never did go alone. Coy wouldn't let me go out on the rock. He was afraid I'd fall and I begged him when he come back up to the top to let me pull my shoes off so I could turn around. He wouldn't do that and I jus' had to hold to the ivy and pull. It's steep now. It's straight up and down. We's huntin' bear grass for salad. It's a great big ole blade of grass that grows over there on the Buzzard Rock. It was tender and it was good.*[75]

In addition to greens and cabbage, Orlean cooked October beans when they were young and tender. October beans that weren't cooked fresh were shelled, dried, and stored for winter use. The dried beans could be parboiled, seasoned, and set over the heat to simmer for a satisfying winter meal.

Green beans were also dried. Orlean sewed these onto strings and hung them around the stove to dry. The dried beans were called "leather breeches." Leather breeches came in handy during the winter months when fresh vegetables were not available. They were convenient, for all Orlean had to do was take down a string of the beans, remove the thread and drop them and a chunk of meat into some boiling water to cook.

Other dried food items included berries, peppers, sage, pumpkins, and apples. To dry pumpkins, they were peeled, seeded, and sliced into circles. Then they were hung on a stick to dry in the house. After drying, the pumpkin rings were stored in cloth sacks.

Apples were dried outdoors. Orlean sometimes used a drying kiln that was located at the smokehouse for that process. But she usually just spread the sliced apples on wire screens and dried them in the sun.

Iduna Quesenberry helped Orlean peel apples for drying:

My aunt used to set with her an' dry apples. I'd go up there an' help her peel apples. Her and Aunt Mary Jane, well they looked for me about every day to come help peel apples. I don't know whether she ever dried any pepper or not.[76]

According to neighbor Charlie Bowman, Orlean dried apples to sell or barter. "In those days people used to dry 'em and sell 'em. That's the way they kept their rations for the winter — dry their apples, put them in a poke and have them to cook in the winter."[77]

Dried apples were wonderful for making sauce, cakes, and pies. Fried pies were made by adding water to the dried apples and cooking them until done. Sweetener and spices were then mixed in with the apples. To make several individual pies, dough was rolled out into circles. The apple mixture was then spooned onto half of each circle. Folded over, the crust edges were then pressed together using a fork. After they were sealed, the pies were placed in a grease-filled iron skillet and fried until golden brown.

There was no shortage of apples for Orlean to dry. Marvin Hawks recalled some of the heirloom apple trees on their property:

There were apple trees all through the property and an orchard across the road. The Paramine apple was good for eating, but not cooking. The Buckingham was a good cooking apple. There was an apple tree behind Aunt Orlean's house called the Smokehouse apple. It was a white apple and good for cooking.[78]

Wavy Worrell remembered the other apple trees on John and Orlean's land:

There was an apple orchard with June apples. It may still be there. At the back of the house, across the Parkway, and in the meadow were apple trees.

One was an "Eliza Jane," another was a June. There were lots of different apples.[79]

Wavy's mother Iduna related an accident she had down by the June apple tree:

I remember she [Orlean] sent me down there [below the June apple tree] one day for somethin' or 'nother." The wind would blow the shingles off the cellar house an' I stepped on a nail. Stuck it in my foot. I came to the house a hoppin' an' Aunt Orlean poured turpentine in the place. When I got home my foot swelled. It was [the] worst sight and I hobbled around for a long time.[80]

Marvin Hawks mentioned that "back in those days they [the mountain people] doctored with kerosene." Marvin and his brother would fetch kerosene from the store for Orlean. The kerosene came in one-gallon cans and the storekeeper would place a ball of candy over the can's lidless spout. He and his brother Everett always ate the candy.

Aunt Orlean doctored with it [the kerosene]. So many drops of kerosene in sugar. Kids got croup and she'd give a teaspoon full of sugar with two or three drops of kerosene. She nursed people. Went wherever and whenever she was called.[81]

Fresh apples were made into cider. Marvin Hawks explained that cider making took place in the cellar house. The cider press was located on the upper level. Apples and vegetables such as potatoes and onions were stored in the cellar house basement.[82]

To make cider, whole apples were fed into a wooden hopper as the cider mill crank was turned. The resulting apple pulp was then pressed until all of the juice emerged. The liquid was stored in wooden barrels and used for drinking. As it aged, apple cider turned to vinegar, which could be used as well.

According to Wavy, Orlean and John had peach trees, too. "When John was livin', a preacher came to stay with 'em. John went to get peaches so Aunt Orlean could make a pie for him." Wavy laughed and said, "Well, John fell out of the peach tree."[83]

Fortunately, John sustained only minor injuries from that fall.

By mountain standards, with their bounty of fruit orchards, vegetable gardens, livestock, and a comfortable home, John and Orlean were living well. With chores to tend and meals to prepare, Orlean's days must have been full, or so it would seem. Little did she know that a new and exciting venture that would take precedence over her daily routine was waiting, just around the corner, for her.

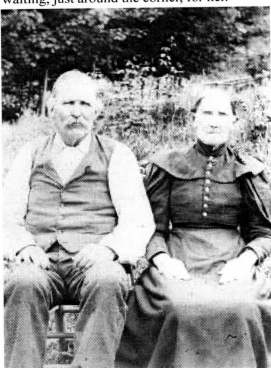

John and Orlean

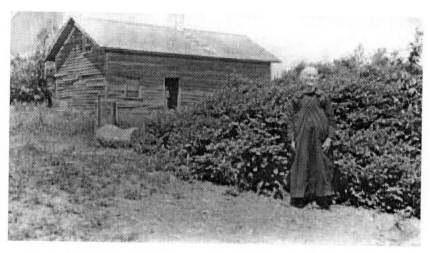

Aunt Orlean in front of her home on Groundhog Mountain

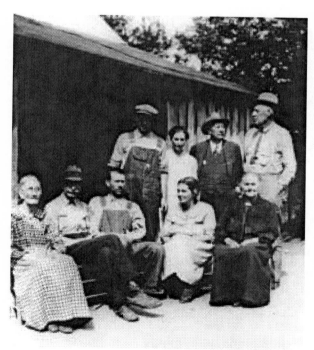

Family Photo: Seated left to right: Aunt Orlean, Eli Hawks, Kenny Hawks, his wife May, Elizabeth Hawks. Standing left to right: Coy Hawks, Lula Hawks, George Puckett, Stewart Puckett

Aunt Orlean's great grand-niece Lossie Viola Puckett with her parents Etta and Arthur. Lossie died from complications of the flu when 12 years old

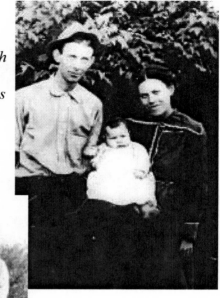

Aunt Orlean's great-nephew Coy Hawks and his boys Marvin and Everette

Marvin and Everette Hawks beside Aunt Betty Puckett's cabin

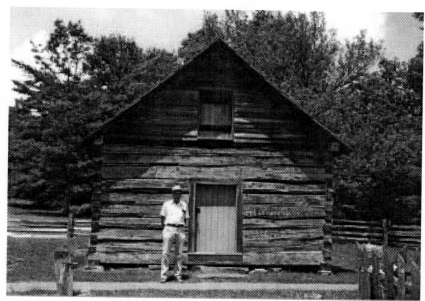

*A grown Marvin Hawks in front of
Aunt Betty's cabin along the Parkway*

*Aunt Betty's cabin was incorrectly identified by some
as the home of Aunt Orlean*

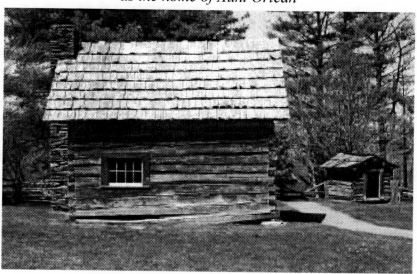

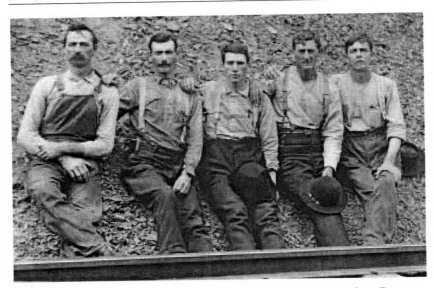

Left to right: Alfred Hawks, Kim Hawks, Kenny Hawks, George Hawks, Posie Hawks. Photo taken in West Virginia (Aunt Orlean's great-nephews Alfred, Kim and Kenny went to W. Va. to work in the coal mines)

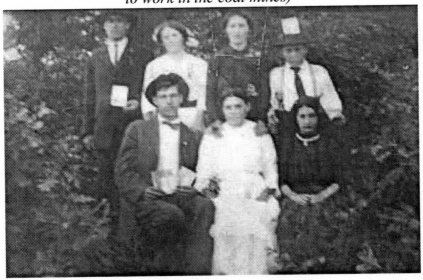

Aunt Orlean's great nieces and nephews:
Front, left to right: Sam, Etta, and Iduna Hawks.
Back, left to right, Kenny, Mattie, Lula, and Coy Hawks

Chapter 6
Midwifery

"She walks the hills by day and night
In all kinds of weather, whatever her plight
Friend of women and giver of life."

—Karen Cecil Smith

In 1889 Orlean Puckett was presumably leading an ordinary and predictable life. With the exception of the changing seasons, each new day would have mirrored the one before. "Alike as burrs on a mule's tail," was a phrase Orlean used to describe her days.

She had a loving husband and family, dear friends, a beautiful home, and, except for an occasional bout of colic and dry eyes, good health. But, she must have sensed that something was missing from her life. The loss of 24 babies would have left a void that ached to be filled.

In the late 1800s there were few doctors to care for the people of Carroll and Patrick counties. Dr. Sawyer, a firm believer in the medicinal qualities of herbs, made his mountain rounds by buggy or on horseback. No doubt, he was thankful for granny women like Jane Hendrick who, at the age of 57, delivered most of the babies in the area.

Marvin Hawks never knew Granny Jane Hendrick, but he did recall a midwife named Ellen Hendrick. "They called her Granny El. They were two different women, but both are said to have been midwives. Tiny Quesinberry was also a midwife."[1]

Coy Martin remarked in a 1976 interview that Granny Jane Hendrick was much older than Orlean. The two lived on the same road along the Parkway, about a mile apart. "Well, Granny Jane is buried [at Bluemont Church cemetery]. I was at her funeral an' I don't guess I was over four years old then."[2] Orlean became a midwife after Granny Jane's death.

A mountain doctor was too busy to worry with childbirth. His primary mission was treating sickness. And, even if he was called to a birthing, the distance he had to travel was usually so great that he seldom reached a mother before her time.

Most mountain physicians, overburdened with their vast territory, welcomed the services of the midwife. Poor mountain families could not always afford a doctor's fees and therefore relied on the generosity of a midwife. Payment for a midwife's services was sometimes only a simple "thank you" or a meager offering of food. There was a constant need for midwives in the hills of Virginia.

In a 1976 interview, Mrs. Ellis Bowman declared that there was a shortage of doctors in the mountain region where Orlean lived:

> *There wasn't but two doctors, I don't think, in this entire county or anywheres near here, right over here, at Laurel Fork. Dr. Cundiff and Dr. Branscomb. And they had to ride horses. There wasn't no cars at that time. I think they moved away before there got to being so many cars. I remember seein' Dr. Cundiff. He come to our house. He was my daddy's doctor. He come over there. He got him a new car and it was a Ford. He come a few times, most time he had a horse. I think Dr. Branscomb kept four horses. He had a team of gray horses. I remember seeing him pass our house. Somebody'd be sick or somethin' and they'd pass there. And come up a terrible storm one time.*
>
> *He went to cross a creek up there somewhere, might've been Stone Mountain Creek. It was up, terribly up, and he got into that water and washed his wagon down a piece and these horses drowned. They moved to Galax or somewhere. They didn't stay over there much longer after that.*[3]

Wavy Worrell said there were two other doctors who served the mountain community during Orlean's time. "Dr. Sawyer was in the late 1800s. Dr. Cundiff and Dr. Branscomb were in Laurel Fork around 1903 or so. Dr. Gates was the last one."[4]

In the early 1900s, Dr. Gates road a horse when he made house calls. Years later, an automobile was his primary means of transportation. However, until decent roads became part of the mountain landscape, a horse was the best way to reach isolated cabins.

Dr. Gates employed both methods of transportation and was still practicing medicine in the hills of Virginia in 1939.

According to Coy Martin, most doctors lived long distances from Groundhog Mountain:

> *They wadn't any doctor any closer 'n Mount Airy, you know, or Winston-Salem, or Roanoke. They'd have to ride in on horses when they did and there wasn't jus' no way to get 'em in. Take too long. Folks 'ud die before you get a doctor in the country.*[5]

Rather than send for a doctor, mountaineers usually called on the local midwife whenever a family member fell ill. She could reach their homes quickly and was knowledgeable of folk remedies and cures. Even though a midwife couldn't administer medicine or perform surgery, she filled a gap that existed in the mountain community's health care system.

It is little wonder that mountain doctors and families held midwives in such high esteem. Their prominence has been recognized throughout the ages. Famous Athenian philosopher Socrates' mother was a midwife. The wife of Pericles, an Athenian statesman and "father of democracy," was also a midwife. Greek philosopher Aristotle spoke of the intelligence and wisdom of the midwives of Greece.

Louise Bourgeois, France's most famous midwife, was born in 1553. She enjoyed a reputation as a great teacher, author, and midwife to the Royal Court for 27 years. King Louis XIII and six children of King Henry IV were delivered by Bourgeois. Madam Le Boursier Du Courdray, another French midwife, went into the provinces and gave free instruction to midwives, using a life-size mannequin to demonstrate delivery techniques. Marie Duges, who was also a French midwife, practiced during the French Revolution.[6]

Justine Siegemundin, Court Midwife to the Electorate of Brandenburg, wrote a text on midwifery that was published in 1776. Eventually, her text was translated into Dutch and used in German universities. Siegemundin was known as a "lantern-bearer in the darkness of ignorance and superstition".

The first English midwife to write a book on midwifery, which was published in 1671, was Jane Sharp. Another book, "The Domestic Midwife," was written by Margaret Stevens, who delivered Queen Charlotte.

Although Florence Nightingale is usually only remembered for her nursing career, she showed an interest in midwifery by writing a book on the subject. One of her nurses went on to found the English Midwives Institute in 1881.

Elizabeth Phillips came to America in 1719 under a commission as a midwife granted by the Bishop of London. Other famous American midwives include: Elizabeth Smithson of Guilford, mother-in-law of the great cleric-physician Jared Elliot; Mary Breckinridge, a Scottish-born nurse-midwife who was widely recognized for her roll in the creation of the Frontier Nursing Service in the mountains of Kentucky; and Quaker midwife Anne Hutchinson. Pastor John Cotton praised Hutchinson for her good works.

To honor her, a statue was erected in front of the General Court of Massachusetts and a memorial plaque was placed in the First Church of Boston.[7]

Some of the first writings about midwives can be found in the Bible book of Genesis. When Rachel was having great difficulty in childbirth, the midwife reassured her and told her not to be afraid.

Later, in the book of Genesis, there is a passage about Tamar, who gave birth to twins. In those days great importance was placed on the firstborn child. During the birth of Tamar's twins, one child put out his hand and the midwife cleverly placed a scarlet thread around his wrist and announced that he was the firstborn. The baby drew back his hand and his brother came out.

Perhaps the most well-known writing about midwives is found in the Bible book of Exodus. The story unfolds that the king of Egypt, threatened by the growing Israeli population, ordered two midwives named Shipharah and Puah to kill all Hebrew baby boys that were born. They were to watch the women while they were on the delivery stool and, if the baby was a boy, they were to kill him. Instead, the midwives lied to the king. They said that the Hebrew women always gave birth so quickly that they never arrived in time. As a result of their courage and loyalty to God, they were blessed with families of their own. The Israel nation was also blessed and continued to thrive.

Known in France as a "Sage Femme," in Denmark as a "Jordemoder," in Hawaii as a "Pale Keiki," in Israel as a "Vartsfroy," and in mountain regions as a "Granny Woman," the midwife was one of the most important persons in a community. She relied on common sense and sometimes employed the use of herbs in her practice. Midwives, unlike most doctors, were dependable, nurturing, and reassuring. They seemed to hold a spiritual sisterhood with the birthing mother.

Wavy Worrell confirmed that Orlean Puckett's midwifery career was born out of necessity. According to Wavy, when no other midwife was available, Byrum Bowman, a neighbor who lived just east of the Puckett's on the Groundhog, sought out Orlean to attend his wife, Laura. Perhaps he'd heard that Orlean had given birth to 24 babies. That fact alone would have been reason enough for Bowman to believe that Orlean knew something about "catching babies."

On that night in 1889, Orlean Puckett delivered her first baby. To Orlean, the birthing must have been like a healing to her soul, for she had discovered her calling.

Wavy commented that McKinley "Kinney" Bowman was the first child Orlean delivered. She went on to explain Bowman's fate after he reached adulthood. "He killed a man named Lee Duggins outside Rome Church in Carroll County. They said the fight was over a girl."[8]

As the legend goes, Kinney had gotten word that his baby sister was planning to elope with Duggins. Set on stopping the union, he approached Duggins on the church grounds where the young men of the community often congregated, sometimes drinking, while the women folk worshiped inside.

According to Larma Puckett, young men waited outside churches just to get a glimpse of the girls. Larma noted that lots of fights happened outside of churches.[9]

After Bowman approached Duggins, the two argued. Shots rang out, and Duggins fell to the ground.

"He served some time," said Wavy Worrell, "then moved to West Virginia where he got shot and killed."[10]

After that first delivery, Orlean became known as a midwife. She went on to secure a worn brown leather doctor's bag, which most likely was donated to her by one of the local doctors. In the bag she kept scissors, twine or string, eyedrops, gauze, and camphor.

According to Wavy, when Orlean "birthed a baby, she gave the child a mixture of catnip tea and sugar to drink before the mother got milk. Comfort plant was made into a tea and used for lots of things. Aunt Orlean used it to cure a baby of pneumonia. There was a plant used to cure rheumatism — hycomtaine. Was a big plant. Looked like tobacco with broad leaves."[11]

"Aunt Orlean used peach brandy in her deliveries and for colds," noted Foy Hawks. "She carried a doctor's bag." Foy pondered over the contents of the bag and said that it most likely held carbolic acid, scissors, and whiskey,"[12] while Marvin Hawks vowed that Orlean used apple brandy. "Billy Hawks would send her a bushel of apples once a year and in that bushel would be a can of brandy."[13]

Orlean's medical bag was off limits to children. Great grandniece Lottie Marshall laughed and said "Aunt Orlean carried a doctor bag or satchel that all of us kids longed to look in."[14] Great grandniece Hattie

Puckett lamented that "Aunt Orlean never let us look in her doctoring bag, but they said she kept eye drops to put in the babies' eyes. Health Department required it. It was a syphilis preventative."[15]

In 1918 the Virginia legislature passed the first law in the state which recognized the midwife. Under this law there were two requirements of the midwife. The first was that a birth be reported within ten days to the local registrar. Hattie Puckett verified that Orlean got someone to turn in the information for birth certificates:

> *They were mailed to the parents. She made a lot of calls with Dr. Gates and he fixed some of the certificates. When we [Hattie and her sister Libby] were born, we got a birth certificate and Aunt Orlean birthed us.*[16]

The second requirement of midwives was to obey the Sanitary or Safety Rules of the State Board of Health. This included the application of eye drops. *Help for Midwives*, a pamphlet issued by the Virginia Bureau of Vital Statistics in 1924, stated:

> *Blindness from birth is caused by inflammation of the eyes caused by disease germs getting into the eyes from the birth canal of the mother, or from her bowel movement. The State law now requires midwives and doctors to put two drops of a one percent solution of nitrate of silver into each eye of the baby as soon as it is born. These are furnished without cost by the Bureau of Vital Statistics, Richmond, Va., to every midwife who asks for them.*
>
> *They are put in wax ampoules with directions in the box. You can pull the eyelids apart easily with a bit of clean cloth around the finger. There is a fine for not using these drops. Do not ask the mother if you may use the drops, the law says you*

must do it. A little redness of the eyes may be noticed for a day or two after, but it does no harm. You are liable to have your permit taken from you if you do not use the drops, or if you make an inside examination with your finger. Call a doctor at once if creamy pus comes from the eyes.[17]

With her doctor's bag in tow, Orlean Puckett would have looked the part of a typical mountain midwife. Although she didn't smoke a pipe or chew tobacco like Granny Jane, she dressed in much the same manner. Most people remembered her as wearing a black bonnet and black clothing. Her long dresses were edged with a "flounce" or ruffle. Wool yarn stockings, held up at her knees with knitted "rounds" or garters, warmed her legs. Beneath black hand-stitched bonnets or scarves, Orlean kept her long gray hair pulled into a neat bun. In cold, windy weather she was sometimes seen with a scarf tied securely over her bonnet and a black shawl draped around her shoulders. When she got old, Orlean walked with a cane and wore tiny, wire-rimmed spectacles.

Wavy Worrell commented in more detail on Orlean's attire:

Aunt Orlean's everyday dresses were mostly solid black, but some were cotton check, full and long, and she called them coats. Sometimes she wore a woven linsey dress and black patent leather belt to church. Never wore panties or bloomers. Wore linsey petticoats and called them shirts. They had a double yoke and buttons down the front. She worked the prettiest buttonholes.

She wore waist aprons with a pocket that were different colors, black and white gingham check. Never wore aprons to church. She wore black shoes called Old Woman's Comfort. Sometimes she wore high-topped ones that buttoned on the side.

Never wore any jewelry. She didn't wear nightgowns, wore linsey underdresses to bed and beneath shirts in winter. They were woven out of yarn and cotton.[18]

Neighbors and family remembered Orlean as tall and slim. Even though she didn't weigh much more than one hundred pounds, she was hale and hearty. Wavy Worrell commented that Orlean's hands were large, callused and strong. She was a hard worker and a dependable midwife. Her pleasing personality and giving nature endeared her to many people in the community. It was often said that Orlean was "one of the best women around."[19]

Larma Puckett recalled Orlean's stamina and dedication as a midwife:

> *I just remember her getting up and going. Dr. Gates worked with Aunt Orlean some. She'd go anywhere. Walk up and down the mountain. She'd go and stay a few days. She was very independent. She was out all during the night on horseback. People would bring horses to come and get her. Sometimes they would bring buggies.*
>
> *I've climbed mountains with that woman [when I was a child] and I would think that my legs would just drop off. I just couldn't make it, but she would. She would get out and walk and go up that mountain. She could go up it and when she did, she would take her time, but she never stopped.*[20]

Orlean was known to ride as far as 20 miles on horseback to deliver a baby. Sometimes she rode her great nephew Coy's red horse Roy or Roadie, the old white mule. For some birthings, men fetched her with their own horse or horse and buggy. Most times, she traveled by foot. Walking five miles to a birthing was easy for Orlean.

In her later years, Orlean depended upon Coy to drive her to birthings in one of her nephew Stewart's cars.

"She never failed to go to a birthing," observed Wavy Worrell. "She borne me and mommy. People trusted her more than they did a doctor."[21]

Stories of Orlean's midwifery skills were repeated throughout the hills. Foy Hawks related one such story:

There was a woman being treated for tumors by a doctor who'd just moved to the area. When Aunt Orlean visited her she discovered that the woman didn't have tumors, but was pregnant with twins. Because of the doctor's treatments [for tumors], the babies didn't survive. When the woman got pregnant the next time, she used Aunt Orlean instead of the doctor and she had a healthy baby boy.[22]

Several mothers in Virginia's Carroll and Patrick counties said if a woman ever had Orlean as a midwife, she'd never want a doctor again. Orlean had a way of winning a woman's confidence. Her midwifery record was impeccable, for she never lost a child or a mother during a birthing. If she foresaw any complications with a pregnancy, she quickly sent for a doctor to ensure the safety of both mother and infant.

In a 1976 interview, neighbor Fanny Brady affirmed her confidence in Orlean's midwifery skills:

I would much rather had her than a doctor. She was with me when my children was born. My baby is 44 years old. I had a doctor with part of my kids, but I preferred her to the doctors.[23]

Another neighbor, Mrs. Coy Martin, echoed Fanny Brady's praises of Orlean and said that everybody loved her. "She was just always ready to go when anybody called on her. I don't think she ever failed to go."[24]

Neighbor Raymond Pruitt, who was 75 years old when he was interviewed on July 12, 1976, was delivered by Orlean. He described her as a good woman. Mr. Pruitt's wife reminisced that Orlean "borned" the couple's two oldest daughters:

> *She brought that [doctor's] bag to our house twice. She really had good luck, because you know the doctors loses some that way. The oldest 'un was borned May the 31st, 19 an' 29 an' the other 'n was borned June 5th in 1931. Now the doctors come to your house then, but you couldn't get one now. They was around, but see they had to go on horseback a lot o' times, in the buggy or something. An' I reckon they [the mountain people] jus' got adapted to her [Aunt Orlean], so most people jus' called on her. Once in a while they would have doctors. One o' his [Mr. Pruitt's] brothers had 12 children an' I think she borned 'em all except one. He had a twin brother an' sister. I guess she delivered them, too.*[25]

Mrs. Dewey Culler, a lifelong friend of Orlean's, related that Orlean delivered some of her siblings:

> *She borned the youngest one. Everyone trusted her with that. And she was with me with all of mine but one. We would go get her and take her back. She would come and stay a few days before [the birth]. She always left right afterwards. I think she was a real good woman. She wouldn't charge us either, but we would always give her a little somethin'.*[26]

The law passed by the Virginia legislature in 1918 required midwives to register their names and correct mailing addresses with the local registrar of the district, city, or town in which they lived. Upon doing so, they received from their local registrar a midwife permit, which was signed by the state and local registrars, which allowed them to practice midwifery anywhere in Virginia. There was a stipulation that prevented midwives from practicing in certain Virginia cities that had regulations of their own. The midwife permit allowed them to charge for their services. The law did not prevent neighbors or friends from attending a woman, but it did prevent them from charging for their assistance. Because Orlean never asked for money, she was not required to register in her district as a midwife. She did, however, apply drops to the babies' eyes and report births, as sanctioned by law. This allowed her to continue helping those who were unable to pay for the services of a doctor or another midwife who charged a fee.

Most people Orlean helped insisted on giving her a token of their appreciation. Raymond Pruitt said that "She never did get no money. People gave her things like food."[27] She accepted corn, beans, hog meat, fatback, cabbage, honey, and dried apples as payment for birthing babies. Other items she received included coffee, ginger, and dresses. Coy Martin said that Orlean sometimes requested broom straw, which was used to stuff mattresses, in exchange for her services:

> Now, when Sylvan [my brother] was born, I
> was a great big boy then. I can recollect that very
> well. She [Orlean] had run out o' straw to go in
> her straw ticks. You know, they had straw ticks to
> go on the beds. Well, that straw'd wear out after a
> while. My Daddy had a stack with some, had some
> rye thrashed out there an' she charged him a load
> o' straw fer grannyin' Sylvan. I musta been nine or
> ten years old.[28]

It was not unheard of for a family to hand over a live chicken to Orlean after she delivered a child. Larma Puckett said that she got a kick out of watching Orlean come in from a birthing, carrying a live chicken under her arm. Although Orlean never asked for money, Larma said that occasionally folks would be generous and slip her five dollars.[29]

Iduna Quesinberry believed the only money Orlean ever received for a birthing was two or three dollars.[30] For the most part, mountain families were poor. Mrs. Ellis Bowman explained the economic situation that existed:

> *There wasn't much money at the time. And, back in those days, people worked all day for mighty little. Some had to take their pay in corn, or beans, or whatever they could, you know, whatever they needed.*
>
> *There was a few people who was a little more wealthy than others. They would pay Orlean or pay people for the work they hired done, maybe a little money. But she, Aunt Orlean, hardly ever got any money. Just once in a while, people would pay her.*
>
> *I think it was a whole family, I believe it was nine in the family, and she never got a penny. Not one penny for going there, and she went there when every baby was born. They just give her a mess of a little somethin' once in a while, a mess of meat. They'd kill a hog. . .and that was all she ever got [from that family].*[31]

Mrs. Coy Martin agreed. "She took whatever they give her, you know. She didn't charge. She went to some of the poorest of families that she got nothin'."[32]

Orlean did not become a midwife to make money. Instead, she simply enjoyed helping others. "I don't think there was ever a doctor enjoyed going as much as she did," observed Mrs. Ellis Bowman. "She had good luck with everybody. She said a lot of times she wished she had a kept a account of how many babies she had borned, but she didn't."[33]

Orlean Puckett's generosity was known throughout the hills of Patrick and Carroll counties, as Lackie Pruitt testified on August 10, 1976. "She saved people a lot of money in this country [area]. She saved them a lot of doctor bills; it would be in this day and time. Pity [that she couldn't be here] today. Cut these doctors out, wouldn't it?"[34]

About a year after Orlean delivered her first child, Kinney Bowman, she went to the home of yet another poor mountain family and delivered a baby boy who, in adulthood, would also become well known throughout the region. But, unlike the first one she delivered, this one would be remembered for his good works. He was the son of Babe and Frances Childress. His name was Bob.

In Richard C. Davids' book *The Man Who Moved a Mountain*, he writes of Bob Childress' account of his own birth:

> *I was born on the night of January 19, 1890. A real old-timey mountain blizzard was howling across the mountains. My oldest brother Hasten was fourteen, and he ran down the mountain to tell Aunt Orlean Puckett that Ma's time had come. Aunt Orlean was a granny-woman, a tall, rawboned lady who was the only sort of doctor we knew. She threw a shawl around her shoulders and set off with Hasten up through the drifts. To Aunt Orlean, every baby was a miracle of God, and folks in The Hollow said she'd never lost a one – though she'd birthed at least a thousand – or a mother, either. I don't know for sure. Anyway Ma was peaceful when she saw Aunt Orlean come in the door.*[35]

Orlean Puckett was never one to let a little snow stop her from catching a baby. Whenever the ground was slick and icy, she'd been known to drive nails through the soles of her shoes to achieve proper footing.

Childress went on to speak of another time when Aunt Orlean came to the aid of his mother. The nine-year-old had developed pneumonia after walking five miles to school in a snowstorm:

> *That night I took pneumonia, and for nine days I was out of my head. Ma held me in her arms most of the time, for she knew how hard and lonely*

a straw tick is to a sick child. Aunt Orlean came to spell her off. I still remember puzzling even in my delirium why she too should care so much about someone who wasn't even kin. I knew we never paid her, and a lot of others didn't either. She'd come when she was needed, no matter what time of night, even if a storm was crashing through the mountains, toppling trees across the path — sometimes for five, even ten miles by lantern light, or up some hogpath that would have made the stoutest man puff.[36]

Every human life was important to Orlean Puckett. She thought nothing of trekking up and down mountains through storms and blizzards, often risking her own life, to help those in need. As a child, Bob Childress had questioned Orlean's selfless nature. Years later, he would apply those same principles to his life as he served his fellow man.

Ninevah J. Willis wrote of Bob Childress:

He pastored six churches located within a twenty-mile radius in three counties: Patrick, Carroll and Floyd. Each church edifice has been remodeled and rebuilt using native stones from adjoining fields, thus making them beautiful architectural structures which blend harmoniously with the rustic hills and the hill people.

They stand today as testimonial monuments to a Hillbilly preacher, a champion among champions."[37]

After the birth of Bob Childress, Orlean continued to act as the community midwife, delivering many mountain babies. On May 18, 1892, she experienced a milestone in her midwifery career. She was called to attend a birthing down by The Hollow at the home of Doc and Nancy Puckett. On that day, she delivered two baby girls. Their parents named them Kelsie Merritt and Elsie May. That was the first set of twins Orlean delivered, and she was overjoyed by the experience.

When Orlean Puckett first became a midwife in 1889, she was 45 years old and her husband, John, was 51. John must have been an exceptionally understanding man, for Orlean was away from home quite a lot during the next 23 years of their marriage.

Midwifery was a fulltime job for Orlean, as explained by Iduna Quesinberry:

> *They kept her busy goin' around bornin' babies. She borned me one morning. I heared 'em tell it lots o' times. Borned me one morning, went below the mountain, borned another youngun, come back an' got her dinner after that. She borned five generations."[38]*

Bell Puckett, who was 90 years old at the time she was interviewed in 1976, remembered Orlean's demanding schedule. Mrs. Puckett said that Orlean would travel below the mountain anytime of the night, riding horseback or walking. She usually went to the home of an expectant mother two or three days before the due date to get ready for the birthing.[39]

In 1912, after Orlean had been a midwife for 23 years, John became sick. Wavy Worrell relayed what she was told about John's illness. As he lay on his deathbed, friends and family gathered in the kitchen. Upon hearing the sound of a door opening then closing in John's bedroom, someone got up to check on him. He found John alert, but alone. "The Lord just came to see me," whispered John, "and he had a bowl that looked like it was filled with moonshine. I'll be using that shortly."[40]

It wasn't long after that incident that John died on March 30, 1912. The cause of death was consumption. His funeral was conducted by Primitive Baptist Elder Matt Blansett and his body was laid to rest in Puckett Cemetery, adjacent to the family cemetery where four of his 24 children were buried. John was just two months short of his 74th birthday. Orlean was 68 years old. The couple had been married for 52 years.

Together they had endured war, hard mountain winters, and the deaths of 24 children.

John and Orlean shared a bond that could not be broken by death. Left alone in her cabin on Groundhog Mountain, Orlean mourned the loss of her husband.

After John's death, Orlean couldn't get used to living alone. It must have been some comfort to her that her sister-in-law was within shouting distance, but by that time Betty was around 85 years old.

Nieces, nephews, and other family members started staying with Orlean from time to time to keep her company. As more birthing calls came, she found herself spending nights, days, and sometimes weeks away from home. Often she'd go ahead days before a birthing and remain as long as a week afterward just to care for the mother and infant. It wasn't unusual for her to leave the home of a new mother and head straight to another birthing.

When Orlean felt overwhelmed by all the demands placed upon her, she'd escape to the home of her neighbors, the Bowmans. Charlie Bowman confided that their home was Orlean's sanctuary:

> *Aunt Orlean used to come out here and visit my mother when she got tired of people coming after her. I heered her come in and say, "Well, I'm plumb wore out and I have to come stay a little while so I can get a bit of rest." Called this home out here. She'd come home to rest. She'd jest get worn out, you know.*
>
> *People would come at all times of the night to get her and take her here, yonder and about. She went everywheres, you understand what I mean, through the neighborhood. And, back in them days, sometimes people had a horse and would ride, but sometimes she had to walk. She'd be on the go from place to place so much and for so long she'd*

*be wore out and wouldn't want to go nowheres else.
She'd jest drop off out here and nobody would know
where she wuz for a day or two.*

*Aunt Orlean was a mighty good old woman.
She went in sickness and birth lyin'. She had a
record of that all over the country. I don't see how
the old lady got around like she did. It's a wonder
she hadn't a got hurt. Now that's the truth. And
they'd take her out all times of night and as old as
she was a getting' and all, I don't see how she was a
getting' around.*[41]

There was an occasion when Aunt Orlean had an accident while
on her way to a birthing. One night, neighbor Walt Allen rode his horse
up the mountain to Orlean's house. Allen's wife was in need of the
midwife. It was a four-mile trip back down to the cabin, and, since
Allen wanted Aunt Orlean to be comfortable, he brought along an extra
horse for her to ride. Orlean stepped up on the tree stump, and, with
Allen's assistance, mounted the horse. The pair made their way down
the rocky ridge, winding through trees and foliage. Halfway down the
mountain, Orlean's horse stumbled and fell.

Orlean was thrown, but landed a safe distance from the mare.
Luckily, both Orlean and the horse sustained little injury and were able
to complete the final leg of their journey.

Two days later Orlean returned from the birthing. She spread
the story of her frightening fall throughout the neighborhood. When she
related the mishap to friends and family, she was quick to add, "If the
good Lord hadn't been with me I'd a been killed." One neighbor made
a joke of Orlean's revelation, laughed and said, "Well, that's the first
time I knowed the Lord looked like Walt Allen."

No doubt Orlean Puckett heard about that joke and, given her
playful nature, probably joined in on the laughter. According to friends
and family, Orlean was blessed with a self-deprecating sense of humor.
She loved to laugh and to make others laugh. She was kind and loving

and never met a stranger. If someone said something against her, she was always ready to forgive.

"She was a jolly old thing, a joy to be around," observed Wavy Worrell.

> *She had a good sense of humor. Wavy Montgomery told me the other day that Aunt Orlean said, 'I don't have but two teeth, but thank the Lord they both hit together'. And another thing, one time Mattie was goin' to the store to take a basket of eggs. Aunt Orlean got out some eggs to add to the basket and said, "Now, tell the clerk between six and a half dozen of these eggs is mine."*[42]

"That ole woman could spread that mouth wide when she got to laughin," Coy Martin mused. "She could laugh as big an' loud as any of us."[43]

Unfortunately, Orlean was very gullible. Icy Vass commented that after Orlean was old and feeble, kids were always playing tricks on her. However, she never got upset.[44]

Etta Hawks, Orlean's great niece, and her friend decided to play a trick on Orlean. There was an expectant, unmarried woman who lived on the mountain. Babies of unwed mothers were called "briar patch" children or those born on "the other side of the blanket." Etta and her friend decided to play a joke on Orlean which involved the unmarried woman.

The two young girls were at Etta's house for a sleepover. Late that night, they gathered up some men's clothes and threw them out the window, then crawled out into the snow-covered yard. Betty's cabin was empty, so they went there to change from their nightgowns into men's britches, coats, and hats. With lantern in hand, they made their way to Aunt Orlean's house.

They banged on the door and roused Orlean from sleep. When she opened the door, the old lady saw two men standing before her.

One of them explained that they had come to take her to the unwed woman, who was in labor.

Orlean dressed, took her bag, and followed the men through the snow. About halfway to the woman's home, the girls started feeling guilty about their prank and revealed their identity. On the way back home, Orlean threatened to whip the girls for bringing her out in the middle of the night. In the end, Orlean softened and joined them in a good laugh.

In 1924, another lady named Fanny, who lived on the Parkway, was expecting a baby. A young man named Russell Puckett knocked on Aunt Orlean's door in the dead of night and told her that Fanny's time had come. He was there, he said, to take her to the mother-to-be. Aunt Orlean dressed, prepared her bag, and left with Russell. When they arrived at Fanny's, Russell told Orlean to go on in and he would wait outside. There were no lights burning in the cabin, but Orlean knocked on the door. After some time Fanny and her husband Isaac appeared at the door, dressed in their bedclothes. "Aunt Orlean! What in the world are you doing out at this time of night?" asked Fanny. Orlean laughed, for she knew that, once again, she'd been tricked.

Even after Orlean reached old age and her eyesight started to fail, she continued to birth babies. Mrs. Ellis Bowman reflected on a night when a man came to take Orlean to the bedside of his expectant wife:

> She used to get in a hurry to go places. One time, I believe it was at some of the Pucketts. They had about nine children. The oldest child, a little girl, she died when she was about two years old, I believe it was. They come after her [Aunt Orlean] one night and it was a little late. She had already gone to bed. She usually retired early. She jumped up and put her shoes on the wrong feet. She never noticed it 'til she got there [to the home where she was going to deliver the baby]. She said she thought

[her feet] felt awful funny. And she just laughed about that.[45]

Larma Puckett, who was a young girl when she lived with Aunt Orlean, remembered another night she was called to a birthing:

She was there when his [Swanson Bowman's] kids were born. They had 11 or 12. He came out there one night and the moon was full. I took her satchel out [for her]. She had eye drops, scissors, and some kind of bandage in her satchel. She got up on a block of wood and then got up on the horse. She wasn't paying attention and got on it backwards. We could see her in the moonlight, sitting backwards on the horse. He [Bowman] started laughing and spitting, and I laughed 'til I cried. I had to sit down.

There she sat up on that horse. She said, "Well, what is wrong with you?"

I couldn't tell her. I just sat there and hollered and laughed. Finally, [Bowman] told her that she was on the horse backwards. Orlean laughed and declared, "Well, I'll just ride this way." Of course, she turned around and rode to the birthing facing in the right direction.[46]

Larma said that sometimes men would come plundering into Orlean's house drunk as skunks. "One man came in drunk and said he came to get her to deliver his wife's baby. His wife was well past childbearing age." Orlean told him to get out of her house and, after he left, she declared that she just couldn't understand why some people had to be so crazy.[47]

When Orlean spoke her mind to men, they usually listened. Icy Hawks related a time when Orlean told a man what to do:

She went to the Martins for a birthing. Aunt Orlean delivered at least 10 of their babies. When she delivered the last one she told the man, "You go

upstairs and sleep tonight. I don't want to come
back here in nine months to deliver another one."
He answered back, "Well, I will tonight, but I'll still
hang my britches on the bedpost." He had a laugh
over that.[48]

Orlean's poor eyesight sometimes caused accidents, as Wavy
Worrell explained:

> *Mommy said she got so tickled one time. She*
> *was up there and Aunt Orlean couldn't see too good,*
> *I reckon, and it was kinda dark in the kitchen where*
> *she was puttin' on bread. She had a little flat, cast*
> *iron pan she was goin' to bake her bread in. She*
> *didn't pour it [the batter] in the pan; she poured it*
> *right on the [eye of] the stove.*[49]

During her midwifery travels throughout Carroll and Patrick
County, Aunt Orlean picked up the latest news. In those days there
were no telephones, so the best means of communication was visiting
with neighbors, hearing their news, and passing it along to others. Larma
Puckett said that Aunt Orlean visited a lot. "She liked to tell all the news
in the neighborhood. Not gossip, just news."[50]

The neighborhood store was an ideal spot to pick up the latest
bit of news. She made frequent trips to the store, and, while she was
there, told what was happening around the mountain.

Lottie Marshall was a child when Orlean called on her family.
She and the other children in the area liked to listen to Aunt Orlean talk
with the other adults. "She visited with a lot of people and knew all the
news." [51]

Aunt Orlean gained a good reputation throughout the hills and
community doctors often called on her to assist them at birthings.
Ninevah Willis cited one such occasion:

> *Dr. Cundiff told me about a time when Aunt*
> *Orlean was present at a birthing. The mother was*
> *having a long labor. Aunt Orlean asked Dr. Cundiff,*

"Is it about time to feather her?" Dr. Cundiff didn't know what she was talking about and he was busy with the mother, so he just answered, "No." But, as the labor went on, Aunt Orlean continued to ask, "Don't you think it's about time to feather her?" Dr. Cundiff finally said, "Okay," at which point Aunt Orlean produced from her bag a goose feather. She stuck it into the fire and then placed the smoking feather beneath the mother's nose. The mother started coughing and sneezing and the baby was born immediately. That practice is called feathering.[52]

Another similar practice that was used to induce a quick birth was called "snuffing." To do this, a midwife held either powdered tobacco leaves or snuff under the woman's nose to produce a fit of sneezing. Herbs, which could be dangerous, were often employed as methods to speed birth. It was believed that Columbine seeds would move the birth along and that Birthwort and Smut Rye would bring on contractions.

To ensure an easy birth, all locks in the house were opened. An axe was placed under the mother's bed and a knife under her pillow to cut labor pains. If the mother developed a fever, a pan of water was also placed under the bed. After the baby was delivered, some midwives made the mother blow into a bottle. It was believed that doing so would help expel the afterbirth and prevent her body from mortification.

If the new mother did not produce enough milk, she was given an herb called Goat's Beard. To stop the production of too much milk, some of it was placed on a hot rock. There were many other superstitions that surrounded childbirth, such as:

A child born at the interval between the old and new moon was fated to die. When a boy was born under the waning moon, the next birth would be a girl. When born under a waxing moon, the following child would be of the same sex. Babies with blue veins across their noses would not live to see the age of 21. A baby born in the morning would see ghosts. If yellow bees were seen before a baby's birth, something good would happen. However, if black bees were seen the news was bad, and meant that someone would die.

Orlean did employ some of the old superstitious ways in her midwifery practice. Great grandniece Dee Spellings recalled a conversation she once had with her mother, Octavia Hawks, about Aunt Orlean:

> Aunt Orlean was an earthy old woman who had a great deal of old wives tales, like putting a knife under the bed [of the birthing mother] to cut the labor. When my mother was carrying Marvin, she went outside to go to the bathroom. She remembered that a sack broke; her water broke. She couldn't see anything that looked like a baby. Aunt Orlean examined her and told her she had been pregnant with twins and the other baby [Marvin] was very much alive. She called the miscarriage a misconception.[53]

Mrs. Willis mentioned another birthing attended by Aunt Orlean:

> A man and his son went to get Aunt Orlean for a birthing. Snow covered the ground and there were deep drifts. They started out in their car [to get her], but could go only so far. They walked the rest of the way to Aunt Orlean's house. Aunt Orlean started back with them, but the drifts were so high they had to pick her up and carry her back to their car and to the birthing. She was pretty old then.[54]

Wavy Worrell had memories of watching Orlean deliver a baby. The mother's name was Susie Ayers, and the birthing took place at Orlean's house. "Susie had her baby girl on the trundle bed," recalled Wavy. "I was three years old."[55] After baby Essie was born, Susie and her husband Bob lived with Orlean for a while.

Mrs. Ellis Bowman pointed out that Aunt Orlean made lots of trips up and down the Groundhog Mountain:

> *I reckon she was on towards 80 years old when she made her last trip down thar and back. Her health begin to fail a little. She didn't take long trips alone. Someone might have carried her down thar. She usually went down to meet them at Mountain View Church on Willis Gap. She went up and down this mountain over here a many and a many of times. She'd go sometimes on a Friday and wouldn't come back 'til about Monday. Sometimes she would be gone a week. [She'd] spend some time with her friends, you know, her neighbors down there. She had a lot of friends. She appreciated them every one.*[56]

Hattie Puckett reminisced about the good times she and her sister Libby had with Orlean and said that they loved her dearly and thought of her as their Granny. The two, who were ages eight and ten, often walked down the mountain path with Orlean when she was on her way to birth a baby. Along the way, Orlean marked the path by breaking limbs so that the young girls could find their way back home. Often when Orlean was away from home for days at a time, Hattie and her Aunt Lula took care of her chickens.[57]

Lula was a favorite aunt who died at a fairly young age. Her nephew Marvin Hawks said that she was around 59 years old when she died. Lula suffered from crippling arthritis. According to Marvin, his family treated her condition with some of Orlean's folk medicine:

> *I can remember going in the woods and trying to find Rat's Vein, a bitter, striped, narrow leaf that runs on the ground, to make poultices out of for her. She could hardly get up and down her knees were so swollen. We were desperate. We felt so sorry for her.*[58]

One time after Lula and Hattie tended Orlean's chickens, Hattie received a reward:

> She [Aunt Orlean] went below the mountain and stayed for I don't know how long. We'd go up there and tend her chickens and feed them. So, when she come back she brought me a dress. I thought the most of that old dress than anything in the world. It was cloth and she'd made it. I can remember that dress just as good. So when she come back, I was at my Granny's. I'd got somethin' in my eye and I was below the house a cryin'.
>
> She asked where I was at and she asked me to come and said she had somethin' for me. When I saw the dress, I stopped crying.
>
> She borned every one of Mama's sisters but one or two. Sometimes she'd walk below the mountain [to The Hollow] and she delivered everybody's babies down in there and she'd be gone for a week at a time. She'd go from one house to the other and stayed that way. When she'd get ready to come back home, someone would bring her back to the top [of the mountain]. Kenny Hawks, Mama's brother, would come up the rest of the way with her. When she got old, friends and family made sure she got from one house to the other when she delivered babies and got her back home safe.
>
> She helped everybody that called on her. I guess she helped to born more [than] anybody around here. She born me and I'm named after her. My name is Hattie Lene.[59]

The name "Lene" was a mountain variation of the name Orlean. Most midwives were so highly regarded by some mothers that they named their daughters after them. It was a typical practice, as in the case of Hattie, to use the midwife's first name for the girl child's middle name.

There was at least one other baby named after Orlean. She was born in Bedford County, Virginia, where Orlean's family lived. On a visit there, Orlean delivered her niece. The name "Orleanie" was bestowed upon the infant. Orlean often visited her niece and family, but when she became old and unable to travel, Orleanie came to Groundhog Mountain.

On one particular visit, when Orlean was confined to the bed, Orleanie begged her aunt to return with her to Bedford. She wanted to care for her and make her last days on earth comfortable. Orlean refused and said that she would never leave Groundhog Mountain. She wanted to stay with the people she'd been around most of her life.

When he was a child, Foy Hawks lived with Aunt Orlean for a while so that he could attend school on the top of the mountain. He remembered the day Aunt Orlean made her last delivery below the mountain:

> *I walked up the mountain with her after she delivered her last baby. We came by a path up Doe Run. There was a rock they call the 'resting rock' and a spring where we'd stop and get a drink of water.*[60]

In 1934, when Orlean was 90 years old, she joined Mountain View Primitive Baptist Church. George Noonkester, was the preacher who baptized Aunt Orlean in the shallow waters of Sisney's Creek, located in Patrick County.

In the baptism ritual, the person to be baptized is led by the hand of the Primitive Baptist preacher down to the water. The water must be from two and one half to three feet deep. "The candidate then turns his face downstream, crosses his hands upon his breast, and gives himself up into the hands of the minister." Before immersing the candidate, the minister states, "In obedience to the command of our Lord and Savior Jesus Christ, I baptize you in the name of the Father, Son, and Holy Ghost." After the candidate comes up out of the water, the preacher declares several times, "Buried with Him in baptism."[61]

Some characteristics of the Primitive Baptist religion include impromptu preaching, line singing, and feet washing. Impromptu preaching means the Primitive Baptist preacher does not use notes or previous meditations in his presentation. It is not unusual for two or three preachers to speak in succession during the same meeting.

Hymns are sung without accompaniment of a musical instrument. The preacher reads the hymn, which the congregation then sings.

The foot-washing ceremony is a somber, sometimes emotional experience and is viewed as an act of obedience and humility. Several towels and basins of water are available for use. To begin the ceremony, someone announces that those wishing to participate should remove their socks and shoes. The washing begins and is done in pairs. Basically, the two individuals wash each other's feet. Foot-washing is not compulsory and is not practiced among all Primitive Baptist churches.[62]

Four years after Orlean's baptism, Marvin Hawks and his family were living with her in the two-story house that John built. Orlean had delivered Marvin and his brother Everett when their parents Coy and Octavia made their home in Aunt Betty's little log cabin. Marvin mentioned that at the time they moved in with Orlean, she was bedridden:

> When we moved down there, she was in the
> bed. Aunt Orlean gave me my first silver dollar for
> carrying glasses of water to her when she was sick.
> I still have that silver dollar.[63]

Wavy Worrell recalled that before Marvin was born, his two-year-old brother Everett would sit on Orlean's lap and run his hand down the front of her dress and say, "Dry cow. Dry as a chip." Wavy said that Everett had heard his elders say that when they discussed Orlean's many pregnancies and how none of her own babies had lived.[64]

On August 30, 1938 Orlean delivered the third son of Coy and Octavia Hawks. They named the child Maxwell and called him 'Mac.' Orlean was 94 years old at the time, and Mac was the last baby she delivered.

Although Orlean kept no records of the number of babies she delivered during her years as a midwife, it is estimated that the figure was well over one thousand.

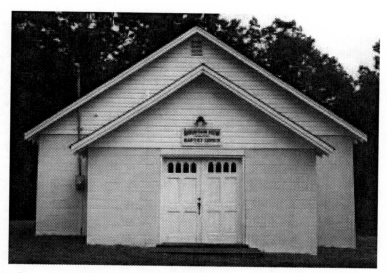

At the age of 90, Aunt Orlean became a member of Mountain View Primitive Baptist Church

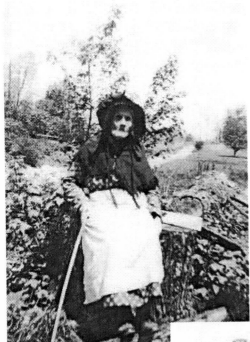

Aunt Orlean

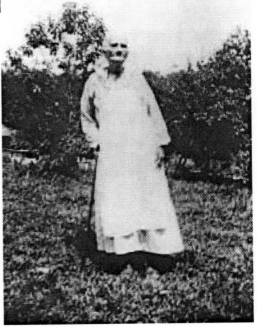

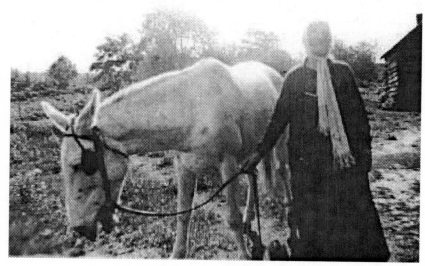

*Aunt Orlean and Roadie, the mule
she often rode to birthings*

*Nephew Stewart Puckett stands by car that was
sometimes used to transport Aunt Orlean to birthings*

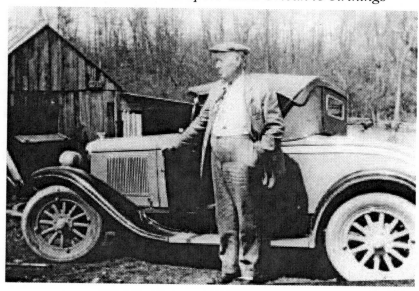

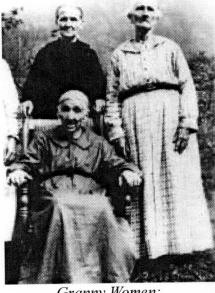

Orlean Puckett with Maxwell Hawks, the last baby she delivered on August 30, 1938

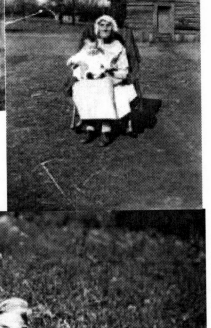

*Granny Women:
Sally Bateman (seated),
Harriet Vass Puckett (left),
Aunt Orlean (right)*

Great grandnephew Maxwell Hawks, seated on "peach seed" coverlet woven by Aunt Orlean's niece "Tilda" Puckett

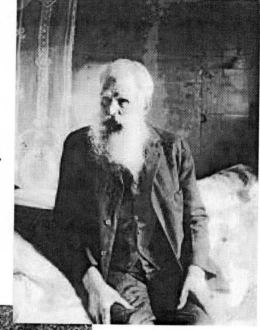

Primitive Baptist Elder Matt Blansett, who preached at John's funeral

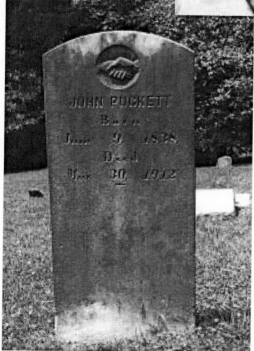

John Puckett's tombstone

Chapter 7
The Blue Ridge Parkway

"My heart's in the Highlands, my heart is not here;
My heart's in the Highlands, a-chasing the deer;
A-chasing the wild deer, and following the roe—
My heart's in the Highlands, wherever I go."

—*Robert Burns*

Shortly after her last birthing, Orlean's health started to decline. She passed most of her days in bed. The woman who had once been such a strong and independent figure in the mountain community was now at the mercy of others. But many of those individuals Orlean had "caught" and cared for over the years were only too happy to do all they could to make her last days comfortable.

Hattie Puckett commented that she and her sister Libby spent the night with Orlean whenever she was sick:

Aunt Orlean never lived by herself. [Her great nephew] Kim stayed with her a lot. Got her wood and carried water. Our mama's sister stayed with her, too. I remember me and Libby both used to go once in a while and stay a night or two with her when she had to stay by herself.

She deeded her land to Kim. He was supposed to look after her, and he did until she got sick. He never married, so he turned everything over to Coy [Orlean's great nephew] so that he and Tavia [his wife Octavia] could look after her.[1]

Although Orlean's health was fading, she must have been comforted by sweet memories of catching babies, of married life with John, and her seven months of mothering little Julia Ann. She had family and friends around her, and, best of all, she was living in the home that

John had built some six decades before. Surrounded by logs John had cut and chinked and items he had carved by hand, Orlean was most likely content in her later years.

She could look out her bedroom window and see the giant blood drop bush where she once hung her clothes to dry and watch the cows and sheep grazing contentedly in the pasture across the road. Old Shep had been a fixture in that pasture, rounding up livestock whenever John gave him orders to do so and Orlean must have thought of this whenever she gazed out her window.

It is not hard to imagine the sights Orlean could see from her bed — a wild turkey leading its young to the spring where she used to draw water; a baby deer wandering so close to her window she could see its faint white spots. She probably heard the chickens clucking and watched as they bathed in the front yard dust. A faint smell of roses would have drifted through the open window and into her bedroom, reminding her of joyous days spent with her sister-in-law Betty. By that time, the old red rambler had grown so tall that it practically covered the front of Betty's old cabin. Betty was gone, but the rosebush she had planted so many years before still remained, just as the house John built. Surrounded by memories of the people and things she loved, Orlean was where she belonged. She couldn't have asked for a more satisfying place to spend her last days on earth. However, unknown to Orlean, a mighty force was at work along the Blue Ridge Mountains of Virginia that would eventually destroy her peaceful home.

Since the early days of the automobile, there had been talk about building a road that would link the Shenandoah and the Great Smoky Mountains National Parks. Such a road would allow a scenic and accessible way for tourists to travel the glorious Appalachian Mountain Chain. In 1933 the National Industrial Recovery Act made the idea a reality. The Act gave the Public Works Administrator the go ahead to prepare a program that would include construction, repair, and improvement of public highways and parkways. The same year the Act was passed, President Franklin D. Roosevelt visited a section of the Skyline Drive that had been built by members of a Civilian Conservation Corps camp in the Shenandoah National Park. A similar route that would connect the Shenandoah National Park and the Great Smoky Mountains National Park was suggested to and approved by the President. By late 1933, $16,000,000 had been allocated for the project.[2]

The scenic highway was a joint project of the Commonwealth of Virginia, the state of North Carolina, and the federal government. While the states obtained land for the right-of-way, the federal government provided the monies. Construction began on September 11, 1935 near the North Carolina-Virginia line. It wasn't until March 22, 1936 that construction started on the 26.33-mile stretch in Carroll County. It would take over four years just to complete the grading work in that county alone. On June 30, 1936 an act of Congress gave the new highway legal status which placed it within the jurisdiction of the National Park Service of the Department of the Interior. The National Park System mandate was "to conserve the scenery and the natural and historic objects and the wildlife therein and to provide for the enjoyment of the same in such a manner and by such means as will leave them unimpaired for the enjoyment of future generations.[3]

Mountaineers had inhabited the Blue Ridge mountains for almost 200 years before the idea of a scenic highway or parkway was introduced to them. The parkway project affected and changed the lifestyle of many mountain folk:

> *Obtaining the right of way involved talking to the mountain people who owned the land, one at a time, on a case by case basis, explaining what the project was all about. For the most part, the mountain people wanted the road.* [4]

To the people of the Blue Ridge mountains, the idea of a new highway meant traveling with ease on a nicely paved road instead of maneuvering the muddy, rutted, and sometimes treacherous paths that snaked down the hillsides. And, most importantly, the highway meant a better and faster way to transport goods to market. Highway construction would also provide jobs and income for many mountain families.

Storeowners would benefit, too, from the influx of tourists the highway was most likely to bring into the area. For those reasons, most mountaineers were in favor of the road. Added to that was the economic situation brought about by the Great Depression:

> *During the Depression, the need to get people back to work was of primary importance. The labor force itself was composed primarily of the local mountain people. About 90 percent of the labor came from the nearby creeks and coves. Only the skilled, specialized labor was brought in from the outside.*[5]

Twenty-five-year-old Floyd Combs began working on the Parkway because the newlywed needed money. "If it hadn't been for the Parkway, a lot of people would have gone hungry in the 30s," he said with a shake of his head. "It sure helped a lot of people out."[6]

Galax resident Dean Higgins had been working for the Civil Conservation Crops for two years, doing landscape work along the Parkway, when he decided to get married.

There was a regulation that CCC workers could not be married. Higgins wed in the month of December, 1940 and left the CCC the following April. A year later, he secured a job on the Parkway, driving a truck and hauling tar and gravel from the mixing plant:

> *I had driven a truck some, but really a bunch of us started driving trucks and none of us had licenses. The state trooper knew we didn't have any licenses, and he sent word he was gonna check on a certain day and we'd better have them.*
>
> *They were doing the license testing here, so I took off and come and tried for a license. I had*

never seen one of those books. He [the Examiner] asked me a couple of questions which I couldn't answer, and then he asked me if I'd read the book. I told him, "no, I'd ever even seen the book." So he gave me the book and told me to go home and study it. I asked him where he would be the next day and he told me Independence [Virginia]. So I went and got my license the next day. In the CCC's I was paid $30 a month plus board and clothes. I got more when I was working on the parkway.[7]

In Fancy Gap, both Mr. and Mrs. Hack Meredith profited from Parkway construction. Meredith worked in the quarry and his wife took in boarders who worked on the Parkway. She kept up to three boarders at a time. One boarder was the quarry foreman, who lived in West Virginia:

He stayed here with us all the time the quarry was running. It was operated about a year. He was the only regular boarder. She charged $1 a day for three meals and lodging. They had to get their washing and ironing done somewhere else.[8]

Workers on the construction project included road engineers, bridge engineers, landscape architects, foresters, contractors, mechanics, masons, power shovel operators, and laborers. Building the highway was a challenge. Not only did it involve moving mountains of monstrous rock to create tunnels and beautiful stone bridges, it also required knowledge and skill to preserve the natural beauty and landscape along the way.

Soil conservation, fire control, erosion prevention, and crop rotation were practices incorporated into the project that made the new road blend nicely into its environs.

Meanwhile, mountain men were earning sorely needed wages. One Virginia man went to work as a grading contractor, making 30 cents an hour. Another drove trucks that carried dirt, gravel, and water to the site. His take home pay for 40 hours of labor was $11.88. A North Carolina man who mixed concrete, dug ditches, and built ramps took home the same amount of pay. The only deduction from their paychecks was 12 cents for Social Security.

Creed Fender of Galax, Virginia picked up rocks, dug ditches, and spread gravel in winter and snow for nine dollars a week:

> *I first helped cut the right of way. I worked at Doughton Park when they were building the park, and I worked some over at Cumberland Knob. I helped do ditching and everything. I just done common labor. I had to walk [to work] part of the time. I walked there, worked all day and walked back. I worked out some awful cold days back then. And I worked on so many roads here and yonder.*[9]

Others worked hard, swinging 18-pound hammers through rock and hand-shaping road banks by shovel. Men were employed to walk backwards, placing stakes along the road's edges every 15 feet. The stakes served as guidelines for pavers. A day's work of placing stakes could cover a span of five miles. In 1937, Fred Handy walked backwards from Deep Gap to Cumberland Knob, inserting stakes along the edge of the road. The distance he covered that year totaled 62 miles.[10]

Some men cut brush and cleared land for the right of way. Later, others sowed grass and worked on landscaping projects. While common laborers were usually paid 30 cents an hour, a skilled jackhammer operator could draw five cents more.

Richard Webb attributed his health problems to Parkway-related work he did in 1937. In that year, he worked in a rock quarry in the Fancy Gap community:

> *I drilled rock in the Meredith quarry with a jackhammer for 35 cents an hour. It was the hardest work I had done up to then and since. There was no loafing. It was dirty work and most of the time after 12 hours on a jackhammer, I would come home*

*and fall into bed. I had no trouble sleeping. At the
quarry, I was replaced by a wagon drill, one that
would pull itself from place to place. After the drill
was brought in, I was assigned to it. I carried steel,
I operated it and did about everything that it
required.*

*One day when moving it, the compressor
built up air and the first thing I knew here come a
hose at me. I grabbed it and it slung me around and
knocked me off my feet. I think that hurt me some.
I'm sure the drilling noise affected my ears. I can
hardly hear now.*[11]

Work on the highway was hard. Temperatures often plummeted
to zero, but construction never ceased because of inclement weather
conditions. Some workers built fires to stay warm.

"We wore our boots that winter in that snow and sleet and cut
dry brush to build our fires with," recalled James Wagoner. "I have took
a gallon of kerosene to start the fire."[12]

According to Fred Handy, crew bosses were stern, sometimes
strategically supervising water breaks so the men couldn't socialize.
Occasionally, blows were inflected upon those who were idle. Handy
described one such boss:

*[He] wouldn't let you gather around the
water bucket for a drink. When the water boy came
around, you had to wait until the man drinking had
finished before you could go over to it. He'd punch
you with a cane if he caught you not working.*[13]

The threat of dismissal usually put idle men back to work. A
North Carolina man who worked on the Parkway remembered one
foreman's repeated threat. Workers carried their lunches in lard buckets.
Frequently, his foreman told those who faltered under the work pressure,
"If you can't git it, git your lard bucket and git!"[14] However, one day the

foreman skipped the warning and fired 40 men because he didn't think they were working hard enough.[15]

Construction was not without risks and casualties. Snakes such as copperheads and rattlers were often encountered along the way, but, from all accounts, there were only a few workers who were ever bitten and none died. Norman Hale recalled seeing plenty of copperheads and rattlesnakes while working on the Parkway. One day, he and some fellow workers ran across an eight-foot long rattlesnake:

> *A couple of them [workers] grabbed them a stick with a forked end and pinned that rattlesnake's head against the ground so he couldn't bite them. Then they kept the snake in an old barrel and covered it up with screen wire. They kept it several days. One day we went to work and the snake had escaped. I was sure happy about that because I was afraid of that snake.*[16]

One laborer cashed in on the abundance of rattlesnakes, offering his fellow workers a dollar for each one they produced. After his workday was over, he'd take his dinner bucket full of snakes to a zoo in Lynchburg and sell them at a considerable profit.

When Calvin Cole worked on the Parkway he also encountered lots of snakes. Cole first worked on the Carroll County section of the Parkway, mainly helping to lay the foundation. Two years later he worked from the North Carolina line to Mabry Mill in Virginia.

"I labored and did a little bit of it all," said Cole, "ran a mowing machine, drove a truck, seasonal work and civil service."[17]

Years later, Cole became a caretaker for the Parkway. It was during this time that he saw a number of snakes, including four or five rattlers. He relayed an incident that happened while he was working at Rocky Knob, next to the Saddle Overlook:

> *I'd cut a tree and was carrying brush out. I just had thrown the brush down. It was grassy and*

growed up and someone hollered, "There's a snake down here!" I remembered then seeing something odd under a rock when I came up. I went back and killed a copperhead. I started back with another load of brush, and there was still a snake under that rock — a rattlesnake. I whacked it with my shovel and killed it. The rattlesnake had seven rattles and a button and was a pretty sizeable snake.[18]

Explosives used in quarry work presented other dangers. While most detonations went smoothly, there was one occasion when a powder house packed with six tons of dynamite exploded. Workers were sent clamoring for safety. Fortunately no one received serious injuries. Norman Hale, who was there when the explosion occurred, described the scene:

I was working in a quarry, using a pick when the boss man started screaming for everyone to run. He said, "Run as fast and as far as you can. A mile won't be too far."[19]

Hale threw down his pick and ran through the woods as fast as his feet would carry him, shielding his ears from the imminent explosion. When it happened, the powder house was rocketed skyward.

According to Hale, the powder house was packed with six tons of dynamite and it [the explosion] left a hole in the ground large enough to place a house inside. The blast was so strong that Hale's wife saw the flash of light from the couple's home in neighboring Galax, Virginia:

When I got home, she asked me what had happened and I told her. Luckily no one got killed, or was even seriously injured. Everyone figured that it was set and that some fellers who had been fired from their jobs had done it. Nothing was ever proved.[20]

Another powder house explosion blew the top off of a Model T car. Earl Lyons, who, along with his brother-in-law Young Anders, worked on the Parkway, witnessed the explosion:

> *I saw the sage grass burning before it ever got to the powder house. It blew the top right off of Jennings' Model T. It just ripped it clean off. That was the only thing it bothered about the car. My brother Charlie Lyons had his lunch bucket in the floorboard of the car and it flattened it. They never did fix Clark's car, he just drove it around without the top on it.*
>
> *They never did find all of their sledgehammers. A lot of the men carried their hammers with them when they took off running out of the quarry. I guess a lot of them just dropped their hammers or threw them as they ran to safety.[21]*

There were other explosions. A jackhammer operator was injured when he drilled into a black powder charge that had failed to explode at the proper time. The accident, which left the worker with minor facial wounds and impaired vision, required a six-week hospital stay. "I almost lost my eyes," said the worker. "I've worn glasses ever since."[22]

While Parkway work was sometimes dangerous, it was always hard. Still, construction of the highway, first called "The Scenic" by locals then officially named the Blue Ridge Parkway, provided many mountain men with jobs, thus rescuing their families from the jaws of poverty. Up until that time, there had been a shortage of jobs in the area. Most jobs paid only 15 cents an hour. Eugene Fortner commented that farm work paid only 10 cents per hour for a 10-hour workday.

Fortner and his father, Garland, drove 30 miles round trip in a Dodge car to work in the quarry. The two used sledgehammers to bust up rocks small enough to go in the crusher.

When an opportunity came along to drive a dump truck, Fortner accepted the challenge. Before securing the job, he had to prove himself worthy by backing the truck into the quarry. He got the job and went on to earn 30 cents an hour for a six-hour shift, which was a considerable salary in those days.

Fortner and his father quit after three months of work because the manual labor was too difficult for his father:

> *I didn't want to quit, but I didn't have a way to get to work once my father stopped going. The work in the quarry with those sledge hammers was real hard, and dad just couldn't keep up.*[23]

Although work on the Parkway was hard, Fortner was proud to have been a part of its construction. He said that the highway proved to be beneficial to the mountain region:

> *It sure is beautiful now. The Parkway put a lot of people to work. There wasn't anything going on in Galax [where he lived] except a couple of factories. Things really didn't pick up around here until World War II.*[24]

Solomon Hawks also made 30 cents an hour working on the Parkway. A month after he and Scioto Sawyers married in 1939, Solomon went to work on the construction crew for the Blue Ridge Parkway.

Solomon's first job was clearing right-of-way. Later, he helped pave the road from Meadows of Dan in Patrick County to Pipers Gap. He also helped build the stone-cased bridge that crosses U.S. 52 in Fancy Gap.

"When they were working close enough for me to walk, I carried Sol his dinner," Scioto reminisced.[25]

Solomon's and Scioto's house, sometimes called the "Judge Bolen house" or the "Mitchell Hotel," was torn down to make room for the Parkway. Materials from the house were given to a man who lived in Carroll County. The man built himself a new house out of the old demolished one.

After the house was completed and the man moved in, he began hearing strange sounds. The noises were attributed to ghosts that haunted the Hawks' house. As the legend goes, four Yankee soldiers who were returning home were captured near Fancy Gap after the Civil War and lynched in the Mitchell Hotel, which later became the home of Solomon and Scioto Hawks. Even after the former hotel was torn down and moved, it refused to give up the ghosts of the Yankee soldiers. Hawks remarked that the man who had rebuilt the house "couldn't live in it because of the spooks, so he burned it. That ended the noises."[26]

Another Parkway worker, Floyd Combs, started hauling dirt for the project in 1936:

> *I worked for about three years for several different contractors. I drove a truck, pumped water out of the holes we'd dug, poured concrete and helped the masons lay stone. I couldn't visualize the Parkway looking as good as it does now. Back then it was just a road being cut through the mountains.*[27]

After serving in the war in 1947, Combs took a maintenance job with the Park Service. "I love the Parkway," he said. "Every day that I traveled it I saw something different."[28]

According to *The Gazette* newspaper, "The Carroll County section [of the parkway] was probably one of the least expensive sections constructed at a cost of $3,271,000, averaging about $142,000 per mile."[29]

The finished 470-mile stretch of Blue Ridge Parkway, surrounded by pristine beauty and rolling landscapes, has given millions of travelers pleasure over the years and will continue to do so:

> *The 300 millionth visitor arrived on August 15, 1981. It is estimated that since 1939 the Carroll County section of the Parkway has been enjoyed by at least 41 million visitors.*

The Blue Ridge Parkway was the first scenic parkway, and it has served as a model for other parkways, not only in the United States but also in foreign nations. The people come to see it and marvel at its beauty and go home with an idea of building one like it. The value of the parkway to the people who visit it is difficult to measure. At the very least, the experience provides an escape from the concerns of their everyday lives. In the highest sense it refreshes the human spirit.[30]

Spring flowers grace the rolling hills in mid-June. By late September, forests are bathed in autumn's brilliant hues of yellow, orange, and claret-red. In addition to a leisurely nature drive, visitors to the parkway can picnic and camp in mountain meadows. Recreational activities include hiking, swimming, canoeing, boating, hang gliding, and cross-country skiing. There are many attractions along the parkway mileposts for everyone to enjoy.

"Visitors to the parkway often remark, 'It's so beautiful because they left the mountains alone.' This is perhaps the greatest compliment which could be paid to the thousands of individuals who were responsible for making the Blue Ridge Parkway a reality."[31]

With all its splendid offerings and a history of providing jobs for the poor, it's hard to believe that the Parkway has a dark side. However, there are those who were adversely affected by its creation. Orlean Puckett is counted among that number.

At its conception, the Parkway was welcomed into the Carroll, Patrick, and Floyd Counties of Virginia. But, as the state began securing land for a right-of-way, bitter feelings started to surface. According to the publication *Mileposts and More*, "much of the land [purchased for right-of-way] had been owned by families for generations and they did not want to sell it."[32]

After the state determined what land it needed for a right-of-way, the property was appraised. Reluctant sellers such as the Powells believed that in order to secure land it was sometimes condemned.

> Sometimes the land would be appraised at below what it should have been. In the case of Laura and Nancy Powell, the part purchased was some of the best farmland that they owned. Laura Powell said that some men came from Floyd, Virginia during the winter when there was one or two feet of snow on the ground to appraise the land. Of course, the land looked worse at this time of year and, since it was covered in snow, just how correct could their appraisal have been? The Parkway finally condemned about 50 acres of their land and paid them $12.00 an acre.[33]

Other landowners like Ann Webb fared some better, but not much. Her family received $300 for 11 acres.[34]

Land was also purchased from the Mabry family under the condition that they would retain lifetime rights to their home there.[35]

In addition to their home, the Mabrys' property included a blacksmith shop and a gristmill. Ed Mabry made shoes for horses, forged iron into tools and utensils and ground bread products:

> From 1910 until about 1925, Mabry Mill was a hub of activity for the isolated mountain Patrick County community. Then the mill's water source, never abundant, slowed to an uneven trickle and Mabry was slowed by a bad back. When Mabry retired, his wife Lizzie took over the milling and many say she was a better miller than her husband.[36]

Mr. Ralph Dexter and his wife, Bell, who lived with the Mabrys for about a year, said Ed Mabry did not want to sell his mill to the Parkway:

*Old man Ed told them he would give them
the right-of-way if they would just go on and leave
him alone, but they wouldn't do that though. They
[the Mabrys] was awful upset over it.*[37]

According to Ann Webb, after Mrs. Mabry's husband died ill
health caused her to move in temporarily with relations who lived five
miles away. Later, when she recovered and returned to her home near
the mill, she found it had been taken over by the Parkway. Unfortunately
for Mrs. Mabry the contract she and her husband had signed included a
section, written in fine print, that stated the house was theirs as long as
it was occupied. Because of her absence, Mrs. Mabry lost all rights to
her home, which eventually was torn down. A log cabin was moved
onto the mill property.[38]

In 1942 Mabry Mill was restored and is now a popular landmark
and tourist attraction along the Blue Ridge Parkway. A gift shop and
restaurant were added to the property. Various demonstrations such as
cider and basket making are presented yearly.

Another family, the Dexters of Floyd County, owned 24 acres
of land located behind Mabry Mill. They planned to build a new home
on that piece of property.

Concerned because they hadn't received a bill for their property
taxes, they went to the Floyd county seat to check into the matter.
Personnel there explained to them that the land was no longer theirs.
Instead, it had become the property of the government and was now
part of the Parkway project. After a court battle the Dexters received
$6,700.00 for the land that was taken from them without their
knowledge.[39]

After the Parkway was built, farmers complained of harassment
by park officials. Since many farmers owned land on both sides of the
Parkway, farm equipment had to be transported back and forth across
the road so the land could be worked. *Mileposts and More* stated that

many times farmers "had to get special permission from the park officials to cross" the Parkway to get to their land. [40]

One disgruntled farmer, who won permission to cross after an extended battle with park officials, retaliated by hitching several trailers and a string of other farm equipment behind his tractor when he crossed the road. His action angered the park ranger, but there was nothing he could do since permission had been granted. The ranger commented that they had not expected him to have a "whole damn freight train!" [41]

The Powell family was reprimanded when their farming equipment tracked mud onto the parkway. On another occasion Laura and Nancy Powell's cattle broke out of their pasture and onto the Parkway. Tourists clamored to take pictures of the two straw hat-clad mountain women rounding up their livestock, but no one, not even the park ranger, offered to help. [42]

To locals, the Blue Ridge Parkway soon became known as "The Devil's Highway" or the "Winding Serpent." Dreams of a hard surfaced road that could be used to easily convey produce to market had not been realized. Instead, all commercial vehicles engaged in business were prohibited to travel the Parkway. Additionally, any vehicles bearing commercial signs were also banned from the highway. [43]

Tourists, too, posed problems. One lady who owned land along the Parkway commented about the tourists: "They'll take your ginseng, pick your strawberries without asking, hunt on your land [and sometimes] by mistake shoot your livestock or maybe you if you're out." [44]

Mrs. Paul Harrell complained that they couldn't keep dogs because the tourists were always taking them. [45]

Another lamented, "City people want recreation, no matter what the expense to country people." [46]

"We had this view long before we had the Parkway and you can't claim it from us," declared a disgruntled mountaineer. [47]

Comments added by others were: "It's the meanest thing that's ever came through here" and "I don't think much of the Parkway." [48]

One man, saddened by the loss of his property, said, "When they treated me dirty like they did, when they took that land down there, sometimes I wished they'd went some other way."[49]

The highway that was viewed by many as a gateway to paradise brought only heartbreak and aggravation to others, as verified by Mrs. Coy Martin when interviewed by the Seasonal Naturalist for the Blue Ridge Parkway in 1976:

> It took 35 acres of our land right here which we could, right now, if we had been able to have kept it, got, oh, a thousand dollars a acre easy enough. Everybody I knew, they didn't like it. Some thought it would be a great thing, but it took our best land, you can see. We all fought it, but it didn't do any good. When the government gets a holt, they gonna take what they want. Oh, if it had jus' been a road, you know, but it took so much of the land. Well, they did do us a little better than some, you know. They offset our house. We're not on the easement an' some are, you know.[49]

Mrs. Martin went on to explain that the mountain people could not use the new road to transport their goods to market, because commercial vehicles were not allowed on the Parkway. The locals did not realize this until after the road was completed:

> It was a slam to us all. [We] couldn't use it [the road]. That's what hurt as bad as anything, you know, because if we hauled cabbage at that time to the top of the mountain, top of Fancy Gap, we had to get on this road up here after lettin' our land go, you know, for this down here.
>
> Folks had to move their houses, but, of course, we all accept it an' get along all right. Oh, there was some completely demolished, tore down on the Parkway. Now, Grandaddy Martin's down

here, he moved his. He moved it back over in the
field where this brick house is here. Course, it's
gone now. Course, we had a big barn right down
here, it was. It was tore down. If you've ever noticed
any rosebushes along the Parkway, why, you would
know there's been a house tore down there.[50]

In 1939, at the age of 95, Orlean Puckett was approached by the State. The highway project was nearing her land, which, she was told, had been selected for right-of-way. Orlean, who was in failing health, didn't want to sell and begged them to let her live in her house until she died. Parkway personnel told her no. Orlean was given 30 days to vacate her property.

Hattie Puckett declared, "When the road come through they pushed her out."[51]

Coy Hawks, who along with his family had been living at Orlean's, began building a new home on property located across the road behind them. Once construction was complete, Coy, his family, and Aunt Orlean moved into their new home. Unable to walk, Orlean was carried from her home of 64 years seated in her favorite rocking chair.

After they had settled into their new home, Coy started tearing the chestnut siding off Orlean's house so that it could be disassembled and transported to their current property. According to Marvin Hawks, his father was going to use the old materials from John and Orlean's home to build a barn on their property.[52]

Those responsible for the aesthetics of the Parkway had decided to keep Betty's tiny log cabin as part of the buyout and preserve it as they had many other original dwellings along the highway. Its authentic and rustic appearance would blend nicely into the theme of the Parkway and give travelers an idea of the way mountaineers once lived. Betty Puckett's cabin would later be marked as Milepost 189.9 and incorrectly identified by the National Park Service as the former home of Aunt Orlean Hawks Puckett.

Marvin explained that Parkway personnel had not been interested in keeping John and Orlean's home, but when they saw the beautiful logs hidden beneath the siding they were surprised. Since it was similar to, but much nicer than, Betty's cabin, they asked that it remain on the property, also. Given, what Coy considered, their callous treatment of his aunt, he refused to let them have her home. He angrily asserted "I'll have cows and horses living in it before I'll let the Parkway get their hands on it." To his way of thinking, they'd already taken enough from his Aunt Orlean.[53]

On October 21, 1939, just three weeks after she was forced to move from her home, Orlean Puckett died. She was 95 years old. Doctor Gates noted on her death certificate the cause of death as mitral insufficiency, but those who knew and loved her said that Aunt Orlean died of a broken heart.

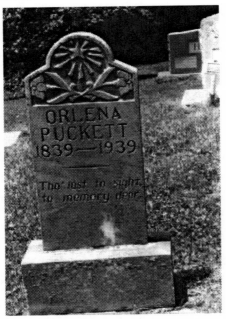

Aunt Orlean couldn't recall the year she was born. Since birth certificates were not issued in Virginia until 1853, the date is hard to determine. However, research points to 1844 rather than 1839 as a more accurate year of birth.

Chapter 8
Journey's End

"Plant you a rose that shall bloom o'er my grave,
When I am gone, when I am gone;
Sing a sweet song such as angels may have,
When I am gone, when I am gone,
Praise ye the Lord that I'm freed from all care,
Pray ye the Lord that my joys you shall share,
Look up on high and believe that I'm there,
When I am gone, I am gone."
—#42 "When I Am Gone," H. M. Turner
The Old School Hymnal, No. 8

At an early age Orlean made preparations for her funeral. Her black burial dress and white hand woven stockings had been neatly folded and tucked away in her pie safe for years, awaiting that fateful day. According to Mrs. Lackie Pruitt, shortly before Orlean's death she changed some of her burial wardrobe:

> Although [Aunt Orlean] was a young woman, she got all of her clothes that she was to be buried in an' she had Mrs. Willis knit her a pair of white hose. She was an old lady who lived on out the mountain here and [Aunt Orlean] kept those hose all the time.
>
> Just a year or two before she died, I was out there one Sunday evening. The granddaughter of this Mrs. Willis, Mrs. Hanks that lives up near Galax, [came by Aunt Orlean's]. She asked her, "If I bring you a pair of nylon hose, will you swap with me?" And she said yes, she would. So, this granddaughter got the hose that her grandmother had knit that Aunt

*Orlean kept for all those years. She was buried in
the nylon hose.[1]*

At 7:10 p.m. on October 21, 1939, the clocks in Coy Hawks'
home stopped ticking. All the mirrors were draped with cloths. The
news of Orlean Puckett's death spread quickly throughout the community.

According to the book *Foxfire 2*, in the mountain regions certain
customs were followed when someone died:

*As soon as a person died, a number of
things were traditionally done almost
simultaneously: a bell was tolled announcing the
death; a neighbor was contracted to produce a
casket (unless it had been made in advance under
the supervision of the person who had died);
relatives who lived away from the community were
notified as quickly as possible— sometimes by means
of a letter edged with a black border; and the body
was washed and laid out in preparation for the wake
that would take place that night in the home of the
deceased.[2]*

Families and neighbors were close. They usually tended their
sick and saw to the intimate details of burial preparation. Seldom did
they seek the services of hospitals or mortuaries:

*Nearly everyone died at home in their own
bed. Neighbors and friends shared in the
responsibility of duties of preparing the body for
burial, making preparation for the funeral, making
the coffin, digging the grave, "sitting up" with the
corpse, conducting the burial service, filling the
grave and placing the flowers."[3]*

After she died, Orlean's body was prepared for viewing. Octavia
Hawks, wife of Orlean's great nephew Coy, bathed her and dressed her
in the black funeral attire. Cloths soaked in soda water were used to

bathe a corpse. Later, after the body was dressed and placed in a coffin, the soaked cloth was placed on the face for short periods of time. Doing this, it was believed, helped produce a more "natural look." Such burial customs were employed before the art of embalming bodies came into being, and, according to Larma Puckett, Orlean's body was not embalmed.

Larma also recalled that quarters were placed on Orlean's eyes.[4] The weight of the coins prevented the eyelids from opening. Silver quarters were preferred over copper coins that had a tendency to turn the skin green. To keep Orlean's mouth from falling open, it is likely that a scarf was drawn beneath her chin and tied over her head.

At the time of Orlean's death, caskets were available for purchase from funeral homes. However, Larma said "Orlean's casket was homemade, made from walnut."[5] It is not known who made the casket, but it was common practice to have one's coffin made in advance. *Carroll County Heritage* states:

> In Carroll County, Virginia until the early 1900s in most communities there was usually one man who made coffins. He kept walnut and oak lumber on hand to make more durable coffins and pine or poplar for the cloth covered versions. He planed (dressed) the lumber in his shop. He kept decorative screws and handle-like ornaments also, but these could be purchased at most any general store.
>
> These coffins were lined with white cloth. The top edge was decorated with fine white lace. Black sateen was used to cover the outside of the softwood coffins (pine and poplar). The more expensive coffins were covered with white brocade velvet. For some, the wood was dressed and polished. Children's coffins were often covered with

*white cloth instead of black. One record was found
which stated that a coffin maker had received $13
for making a coffin for a well-to-do family and he
had furnished all the materials.*[6]

Larma Puckett said that Orlean's coffin was placed in the home
of Coy and Octavia Hawks. According to her, a body was usually
positioned in the parlor, which was a special room set aside for company.
The custom was to sit up with the dead.[7]

All day and night friends and family poured into the Hawks
home to pay their respects to the woman they had loved and admired.
Most who came could boast that they were birthed by the loving hands
of midwife Orlean Puckett. Through tears and laughter they shared
stories of the woman who had made such a difference in their lives and
in the mountain community of Carroll and Patrick counties. They
remembered how well she got along with everyone, how she believed in
equality. One of her favorite sayings was "There won't be separate
stalls in heaven." She would have been happy to see the community
fellowshipping together that evening.

Food brought in by neighbors filled the kitchen table and spilled
over onto the countertops. That night there would not have been a
shortage of volunteers to "sit up with the corpse."

In *Foxfire 2*, Aunt Arie described what it was like before a
funeral:

*Friends would come in, stay all night, bring
food. It was a comfort to th'family in case they
should need anything. Along about midnight, they'd
sing some hymns soft. And they'd stay until th'body
was taken to th'church. Now they sit up all night in
th'funeral parlor, but they still stay with th'body.
Before bodies were preserved, funerals usually took
place soon after the death, often, in fact, the next
day.*[8]

The air was probably crisp and clean on that October day when Orlean's funeral took place. Mourners filled the Hawks' home, flowing out onto a yard covered with the last leaves of autumn.

"I remember the funeral," Larma Puckett remarked. "Everybody in the country knew Aunt Orlean and there was a crowd there. The service was held inside the house and those who couldn't get in stood outside."[9]

Icy Hawks recalled that George Noonkester and Isaac Quesenberry preached at Orlean's funeral:

> *Hubert Hawks, a Missionary Baptist preacher, attended but didn't preach. He knew her well. George was the preacher at Mountain View. He told at her funeral about her working for a quarter a day or a pound of lard.*[10]

George Noonkester was the preacher who had baptized Orlean five years earlier.

After the eulogy was delivered, the song leader stood up and read the first line of a song from the Primitive Baptist hymnal.

"They sang 'When I Am Gone,'" said Icy Hawks. "Sang it out in the yard at Coy's house."[11] Lottie Marshall explained that in Primitive Baptists "line songs" the song leader would read one line of the hymn, then "the congregation would sing it. Song was sung one line at a time without musical instruments."[11]

There has been some speculation as to why songs were sung in such a manner. One explanation is that the practice began in the old days when many people were unable to read. Line songs gave everyone the opportunity to participate.

"Shed not a tear o'er your friend's early bier," the song leader proclaimed loudly so that those standing in the yard of Coy Hawks' house could hear. The congregation responded in song: "Shed not a tear o'er your friend's early bier." And so the line song continued through all three verses, echoing over the hills and into the hollows Aunt Orlean had trod countless days and nights delivering babies, tending the sick, and spreading happiness and love to her neighbors.

Larma Puckett commented that neighborhood men dug Orlean's grave. "There were no vaults in graves then. Her casket was carried from Coy's house to the graveyard."[12]

As her coffin was lifted by family and friends and carried to the cemetery, mourners followed solemnly behind. Across the new road that had caused so much heartache and onto a dirt path dwarfed by hickory, maple, and blackgum the procession made its way. At the cemetery, Orlean's coffin was lowered into the earth beside of John's grave.

"When they buried someone," explained Marvin Hawks, "they had a little house they'd put over the graves for a while. They'd put a little shelter over the fresh grave so it wouldn't wash."[13]

There were no flowers at Orlean's funeral. According to custom, family members often planted flowers on the graves of their loved ones.

Some years later, a tombstone, skillfully and beautifully engraved with a star and two lilies, would bear the words "Tho' lost to sight, to memory dear."

To this day that line holds true, for Orlean Puckett's memory still lingers along the Blue Ridge Parkway, touching the lives of even those who never knew her. After a lifetime of sorrow, joy, laughter, and service to others, Aunt Orlean is finally at rest. And, as Ellis Bowman, a friend and neighbor, once commented, "She's getting her reward now."[14]

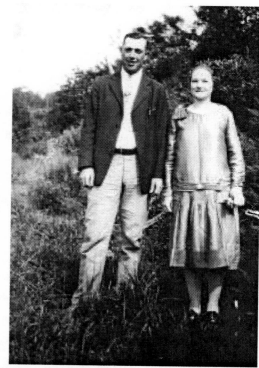

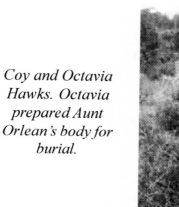

Coy and Octavia Hawks. Octavia prepared Aunt Orlean's body for burial.

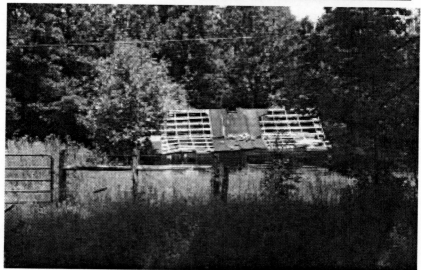

What remains of the house where Aunt Orlean died.

Epilogue

In 1976 nurse-midwives, registered nurses who are also trained as midwives, became regulated in Virginia. A small number of lay midwives or "granny women" who had practiced prior to 1976 and were registered with the Health Department are still allowed to practice in the state. Direct entry midwives are identified as those who are not required to be nurses, who may or may not have a college degree, and who received their education through multiple routes such as apprenticeship, workshops, etc. Direct entry midwives are not allowed to practice in the state of Virginia.

According to the group Citizens for Midwifery, "Direct entry midwives practice legally in 33 states: fourteen states regulate these midwives, most by licensing, and midwives practice without regulation, but legally, in the remaining 19 states. At this time, only 9 states plus the District of Columbia actually prohibit direct entry midwives from practicing by statute or judicial interpretation, and in 8 states licensure is required by statute but no licenses are issued. So, direct entry midwives are practicing legally in 33 states, while they practice unlawfully or illegally in 17 states. However, these figures are subject to change as new legislation is enacted or new legal opinions are established that can change status in the illegal states."[1]

A Virginia midwife who, in 1995, delivered a baby in an isolated Middleburg cabin, was charged with manslaughter 16 months after the infant died. The Loudoun County prosecutor dropped the manslaughter charges after the dead baby's parents could not be located.

The Middleburg mother had insisted on giving birth to her first child in the rustic cottage where she and her husband lived without electricity. Besides the parents, there were two other individuals present at the birthing — a family friend and an unlicensed lay midwife. The birthing was described in an article from *The Washington Post*:

> *"Twenty minutes before delivery, though, on*
> *a cold January evening in 1995, something went*

terribly wrong. The baby girl's umbilical cord became compressed, cutting off blood flow and slowing her heartbeat. But, it wasn't until after the unconscious baby was born – more that 20 minutes after the first sign of trouble – that someone in the house called for outside medical help, according to court records and those familiar with the case."[2]

The baby died the following day. After being tipped off by a physician, an investigation of the midwife ensued and led to a grand jury indictment.

While obstetric specialists admitted that there was no guarantee the infant would have lived had the mother been transported to a hospital, they conclude that the odds would have been much better. The breech birth, they contend, would have been avoided since most babies in the breech position are delivered through Caesarean section.

The parents acknowledged that they knew the risks of having the baby at home. Despite the complications of a breech birth, they decided to go through the birth at home. After the death of their child, they were supportive of the midwife and did not press charges. They have since moved to an undisclosed location.

However, the Commonwealth's attorney has vowed to keep searching for the parents in hopes that the manslaughter charge can be reinstated. If convicted, the midwife could face up to 10 years in prison.[3]

In 1999, a Virginia midwife and her assistant were indicted for practicing midwifery without a license, practicing medicine without a license, and involuntary manslaughter. The felony count of involuntary manslaughter stemmed from the 1997 death of a woman approximately 10 hours after a successful home birth. The mother, whose first three children were delivered by Caesarean section in hospitals, had resolved to deliver her fourth child at home. The 30-year-old was reported to have bled to death after delivering a healthy girl.

More than eight months after the death, an autopsy report, included in court affidavits, stated that the mother's uterus did not properly contract after birth, causing her to suffer extensive blood loss which occurred over a long time and "would have been obvious to any trained or experienced person." The papers also stated that the death could have been prevented if she had been hospitalized in time to receive a transfusion.

A lawyer for the midwife insisted that the affidavits were incorrect in describing the obviousness and the extent of blood loss. He went on to say that even if the woman had delivered the child in a hospital there was no assurance that a blood transfusion would have saved her life.[4]

The midwives' trial was scheduled for January 14, 2000. Proponents in favor of legalizing midwifery feared that the case would harm a bill before the Virginia General Assembly that could lead to the licensing of direct entry midwives.

The trial, which happened to be on International Midwives' Day, ended with plea-bargains. One-year jail sentences and a portion of the fines were suspended. It was a bittersweet victory for the midwife and her assistance.[5]

Along with Virginia and seven other states, North Carolina does not recognize direct-entry midwives. Since 1983, practicing midwifery without a license in North Carolina has been a misdemeanor.

Amy Medwin, Certified Childbirth Educator, Certified Professional Midwife, and Doula was arrested in North Carolina in the spring of 1998 for practicing midwifery without a license.

After assisting at a difficult birthing, Medwin called rescue workers to transfer the infant to a hospital. The child weighed over 10 pounds and was having difficulty breathing. Medwin administered oxygen, but chose to transport as an added precaution. Following a stay in the hospital, the child proved to be healthy and there were no complications.

It was that hospital transport that alerted authorities to Medwin's illegal midwifery practice. However, authorities waited and watched until Medwin attended another birth before arresting her. After much publicity and an outpouring of community support, Medwin's case was dismissed due to a technicality.

Medwin, who began attending births in 1979, received her certification in January 1998 from the North American Registry of Midwives. Prior to her arrest in 1998 she had attended over 600 labors. According to North Carolina law, Medwin has never been allowed to practice midwifery in the state; however, there is no restraining order against her.

Medwin, like many others, would like to see a change in laws against midwifery. According to her, if midwives are legalized, they can work together with doctors for the welfare of the baby and the mother whenever special needs arise or transfer of care is necessary. Until midwifery is legalized in all states, secret births and occasional arrests will continue and doctors will see only the complications, not the dozens of other normal, healthy births.

Medwin believes that women should have the right to birth wherever and with whomever they choose. For many, that choice is a midwife-assisted home birth.

Although Medwin believes in the appropriate use of technology, she said that midwives look even deeper. They do not view childbirth as an illness. They listen to the mother when she expresses anxious concern. They look, feel, and depend on their own instincts. That sets them apart from doctors.

> *"The midwife can't perform surgery,"*
> *Medwin said, "but certified midwives can do*
> *everything else well and understand all aspects of*
> *CPR and carry emergency supplies. Midwives are*
> *well trained in all aspects of normal pregnancy,*
> *labor, and childbirth. They are also well versed in*
> *how to determine when a pregnancy is deviating from*
> *normal and if a consult is necessary. They fight for*
> *the mother and work to help women who are trying*

to conceive and bear children. They form a bond
with the mother that continues as the child grows."[6]

Orlean Puckett experienced such a bond with the generations of women she assisted in childbirth.

Today large numbers of women seek the services of the midwife. Their reasons for choosing a midwife over an obstetrician are varied. For some, medical expense is the leading factor, with a doctor's fee averaging $5,000 and a lay midwife's fee less than 25 percent of that. Others simply want the home birth experience. Most choose the midwife because she offers a quality of personal care and attention that could never be obtained in a doctor's office or hospital. Lower infant mortality rate is cited as one of the major reasons for choosing a home birth midwife.

Midwifery, it would seem, is as old as time. Orlean Puckett and those midwives who came before her were depended upon and revered by many. And, though their sacrifices were great, they did not face the strict laws and regulations that midwives are subject to today. Virginia Statutory Laws identify a midwife as follows:

Any person who, for compensation, assists
in delivery and postnatal care by affirmative act or
conduct immediately prior and subsequent in the
labor attendant to childbirth in conjunction with or
in lieu of a member of the medical profession shall
be deemed a midwife and to be practicing midwifery.
As used in this section, 'compensation' means
anything of value received before or after the labor
attendant to childbirth, with or without an express
agreement between the person so assisting and the
patient or anyone in the patient's behalf.[7]

If she were still alive and practicing midwifery in Virginia, Orlean Puckett, even with her exemplary and impeccable birthing skills, would be subject to arrest and prosecution. Even though she never required money for her services, Orlean was often given money or gifts when she delivered a child. Under Virginia's Statutory Laws on midwifery, this action would have been considered as receiving compensation. To further complicate matters, Orlean Puckett was never registered in Virginia as a midwife, so she would not have been "grandfathered" as one who legally practiced midwifery prior to 1976.

Like many of those who came before her, Orlean Puckett forged a path, setting a positive example for future midwives. Because of her relentless desire and dedication to help women, her name will be esteemed and forever remembered along Virginia's Blue Ridge Parkway.

NOTES

Chapter 1 – The Early Years

1. *Carroll County Heritage, Vol. 1, Carroll County, Virginia 1842-1994*, Walworth Publishing Co., 1994, p. 11.
2. Worrell, Wavy – Interviewed by Karen Cecil Smith, July 11, 1997.
3. Willis, Ninevah J., *Typical Mountain People, Country Living*, private unpublished collection held by the Hillsville Historical Society, Hillsville, VA, p. 7.
4. Willis, *Typical Mountain People*, p. 7.
5. Bowman, Mrs. Ellis – Interviewed by Brenda Bowers August 20, 1976.
6. Haymore, Rev. C. C., *Letter to the Editor, Republican Newspaper*, Yadkinville, NC, September 6, 1900.
7. Hawks, Marvin – Interviewed by Karen Cecil Smith, June 22, 1998.
8. Martin, Coy – Interviewed by Brenda Bowers, September 13, 1976.
9. Worrell, Wavy – Interviewed by Karen Cecil Smith, September 11, 1997.

Chapter 2- Young Love and the Civil War

1. Smith, May Belle T., *The Puckett Family Genealogy – 1998*, pp. 8-9.
2. Puckett, David – Interviewed by Karen Cecil Smith, September 15, 1998.
3. Willis, *Typical Mountain People*, p. 8.
4. Puckett, Hattie – Interviewed by Karen Cecil Smith, May 18, 1997.

5. Puckett, David – Interviewed by Karen Cecil Smith, March 6, 2001.

6. Pruitt, Raymond – Interviewed by Brenda Bowers, July 12, 1976.

7. Pruitt, Mrs. Raymond – Interviewed by Brenda Bowers, July 12, 1976.

8. Worrell, Wavy – Interviewed by Karen Cecil Smith, July 11, 1997.

9. Pruitt, Mrs. Raymond – Interviewed by Brenda Bowers, July 12, 1976.

10. Pruitt, Mrs. Raymond and Pruitt, Lackie – Interviewed by Brenda Bowers, July 12, 1976 and August 10, 1976.

11. Worrell, Wavy – Interviewed by Karen Cecil Smith, July 11, 1997.

12. Worrell, Wavy – Interviewed by Karen Cecil Smith, July 11, 1997.

13. Hawks, Foy – Interviewed by Karen Cecil Smith, April 6, 1997.

14. Worrell, Wavy – Interviewed by Karen Cecil Smith, July 23, 1998.

15. Puckett, Hattie – Interviewed by Karen Cecil Smith, May 18, 1997.

16. *The History Place – U. S. Civil War 1861-1865*, http://www.historyplace.com/civilwar/

17. Croteau, Maureen and Worcester, Wayne, *The Essential Researcher*, Harper Collins Publishers, New York, NY, 1993, p.45.

18. Walker, Gary C., *The War in Southwest Virginia 1861-65*, A & W Enterprise, Roanoke, VA, 1985, p. 19.

19. Strait, Alan, *Brother Against Brother*, http://members.tripod.com/~ALZWIRED/cwone

20. Clifton, Neale, *Regimental Histories of Our Ancestors – Confederate States of America – 50th Virginia Infantry*, http://www.pilot.infi.net/~nkcliftn/csaregim.htm

21.   Smith, *The Puckett Family Genealogy,* p. iii.
22.   Smith, *The Puckett Family Genealogy*, p. 40.
23.   Puckett, David – Interviewed by Karen Cecil Smith, March 6, 2001.
24.   Puckett, David – Interviewed by Karen Cecil Smith, September 15, 1998.
25.   Letter from Hollywood Cemetery, August 18, 1998.
26.   Puckett, David – Interviewed by Karen Cecil Smith, September 15, 1998.
27.   Smith, *The Puckett Family Genealogy,* p. 40.
28.   Smith, *The Puckett Family Genealogy*, pp. 11, 40.
29.   Walker, *The War in Southwest Virginia 1861-65,* p.67.
30.   Walker, *The War in Southwest Virginia 1861-65,* pp. 11,16.
31.   Lonn, Ella, *Desertion During the Civil War,* The American Historical Association, Gloucester, Mass., 1982, Reprinted by Permission of Appleton-Century-Crofts, Inc., 1966, pp. 8, 10, 11.
32.   Lonn, *Desertion During the Civil War*, pp. 8, 10, 11.
33.   Puckett, David – Interviewed by Karen Cecil Smith, September 15, 1998.
34.   Lonn, *Desertion During the Civil War,* p. 12.
35.   Ray, Delia, *Behind the Blue and Gray,* Lodestar Books, Laing Communications, Inc., Bellevue, WA, 1991, p. 42.
36.   Worrell, Wavy – Interviewed by Karen Cecil Smith, April 28, 1998.
37.   Spellings, Dee – Interviewed by Karen Cecil Smith, August 7, 1998.
38.   Worrell, Wavy – Interviewed by Karen Cecil Smith, July 11, 1997.
39.   Haymore, *Letter to the Editor*, September 16, 1900.
40.   Worrell, Wavy – Interviewed by Karen Cecil Smith, July 11, 1997.

41. Kunz, Jeffrey R. M. and Finkel, Asher, J., *The American Medical Association Family Medical Guide,* Random House, Inc., New York, NY, 1987, p. 719.

42. Vass, Icy – Interviewed by Karen Cecil Smith, June 22, 1998.

43. Lonn, *Desertion During the Civil War,* p. 65.

44. Worrell, Wavy – Interviewed by Karen Cecil Smith, April 28, 1998.

45. Puckett, David – Interviewed by Karen Cecil Smith, September 14, 1998.

46. Hawks, Marvin – Interviewed by Karen Cecil Smith, June 22, 1998.

47. Hawks, Foy – Interviewed by Karen Cecil Smith, April 16, 1997.

48. Worrell, Wavy – Interviewed by Karen Cecil Smith, July 11, 1997.

49. Quesinberry, Iduna – Interviewed by Brenda Bowers, July 16, 1976 and July 20, 1976.

50. Willis, Ninevah J. – Interviewed by Karen Cecil Smith, July 9, 1998.

51. *The History Place – U. S. Civil War 1861-1865,* http://www.historyplace.com/civilwar/

Chapter 3 – The Babies

1. Pruitt, Mrs. Raymond – Interviewed by Brenda Bowers, July 12, 1976.

2. Bowman, Charlie – Interviewed by Brenda Bowers, July 26, 1976.

3. Culler, Mrs. Dewey – Interviewed by Brenda Bowers, July 30, 1976.

4. Bowman, Mrs. Ellis – Interviewed by Brenda Bowers, August 20, 1976.

5. Puckett, Hattie – Interviewed by Karen Cecil Smith, May 18, 1997.

6. Worrell, Wavy – Interviewed by Karen Cecil Smith, July 11, 1997.

7. Bowman, Charlie – Interviewed by Brenda Bowers, July 26, 1976.

8. Puckett, Hattie – Interviewed by Karen Cecil Smith, May 18, 1997.

9. Haymore, *Letter to the Editor*, September 16, 1900.

10. Puckett, Hattie – Interviewed by Karen Cecil Smith, May 18, 1997.

11. Information provided by Wayne Rossi, Sera-Tec Biologicals, Chapel Hill, NC, June 19, 1998.

12. Puckett, Shelby, *Aunt Orlena Puckett, Carroll County Heritage, Vol.I,* Walsworth Publishing Co., 1977, p. 236.

Chapter 4 – John and Orlean

1. Bowman, Mrs. Ellis – Interviewed by Brenda Bowers, August 20, 1976.

2. Worrell, Wavy – Interviewed by Karen Cecil Smith, July 11, 1997.

3. Martin, Coy – Interviewed by Brenda Bowers, July 13, 1976.

4. Pruitt, Raymond – Interviewed by Brenda Bowers, July 12, 1976.

5. Worrell, Wavy – Interviewed by Karen Cecil Smith, July 11, 1997.

6. Martin, Coy – Interviewed by Brenda Bowers, July 13, 1976.

7. Davids, Richard C., *The Man Who Moved A Mountain,* Fortress Press, 1970, pp. 49, 50.

8. Puckett, David – Interviewed by Karen Cecil Smith, March 6, 2001.

9. Puckett, Larma – Interviewed by Karen Cecil Smith, July 16, 1998.

10. Hawks, Foy – Interviewed by Karen Cecil Smith, April 6, 1997.

11. Hawks, Marvin – Interviewed by Karen Cecil Smith, June 22, 1998.

12. Worrell, Wavy – Interviewed by Karen Cecil Smith, July 23, 1998.

Chapter 5 – Groundhog Mountain

1. Worrell, Wavy – Interviewed by Karen C. Smith, July 11, 1997.

2. Haymore, *Letter to the Editor,* September 16, 1900.

3. *A Remarkable Woman,* Article in *The Republican Newspaper,* September 16, 1900.

4. Worrell, Wavy – Interviewed by Karen C. Smith, July 11, 1997.

5. Bowman, Nannie – Interviewed by Karen Cecil Smith, July 16, 1998.

6. Bowman, Mrs. Ellis – Interviewed by Brenda Bowers, August 20, 1976.

7. Worrell, Wavy – Interviewed by Karen C. Smith, July 11, 1997.

8. Hawks, Marvin – Interviewed by Karen C. Smith, June 22, 1998.

9. Worrell, Wavy – Interviewed by Karen C. Smith, July 11, 1997.

10. Pruitt, Mrs. Lackie – Interviewed by Brenda Bowers, August 10, 1976.

11. Hawks, Marvin – Interviewed by Karen Cecil Smith, June 22, 1998.

12. Worrell, Wavy – Interviewed by Karen Cecil Smith, July 11, 1997.

13. Puckett, David – Interviewed by Karen Cecil Smith, September 15, 1998.

14. Worrell, Wavy – Interviewed by Karen Cecil Smith, July 11, 1997.

15. Martin, Coy – Interviewed by Brenda Bowers, July 13, 1976.
16. Worrell, Wavy – Interviewed by Karen Cecil Smith, July 11, 1997.
17. Puckett, Larma – Interviewed by Brenda Bowers, July 26, 1976.
18. Quesinberry, Iduna – Interviewed by Karen Cecil Smith, July 11, 1997.
19. Worrell, Wavy – Interviewed by Karen Cecil Smith, July 11, 1997.
20. Puckett, Larma – Interviewed by Brenda Bowers, July 26, 1976.
21. Worrell, Wavy – Interviewed by Karen Cecil Smith, July 11, 1997.
22. Puckett, Larma – Interviewed by Brenda Bowers, July 26, 1976.
23. Worrell, Wavy – Interviewed by Karen Cecil Smith, July 11, 1997.
24. Worrell, Wavy – Interviewed by Karen Cecil Smith, July 11, 1997.
25. Quesinberry, Iduna – Interviewed by Brenda Bowers, July 16, 1976.
26. Hawks, Marvin – Interviewed by Karen Cecil Smith, June 22, 1998.
27. Quesinberry, Iduna – Interviewed by Brenda Bowers, July 16, 1976.
28. Quesinberry, Iduna – Interviewed by Brenda Bowers, July 16, 1976.
29. Puckett, Hattie – Interviewed by Karen Cecil Smith, May 18, 1997.
30. Hawks, Marvin – Interviewed by Karen Cecil Smith, June 22, 1998.
31. Pruitt, Raymond – Interviewed by Karen Cecil Smith, April 15, 1997.
32. Puckett, David – Interviewed by Karen Cecil Smith, September 14, 1998.

33.   Worrell, Wavy – Interviewed by Karen Cecil Smith, July 11, 1997.

34.   Hawks, Marvin – Interviewed by Karen Cecil Smith, June 22, 1998.

35.   Worrell, Wavy – Interviewed by Karen Cecil Smith, May 3, 1998.

36.   Quesinberry, Iduna – Interviewed by Brenda Bowers, July 16, 1976 and July 20, 1976.

37.   Puckett, Larma – Interviewed by Karen Cecil Smith, July 16, 1998.

38.   Quesinberry, Iduna – Interviewed by Brenda Bowers, July 16, 1976 and July 20, 1976.

39.   Quesinberry, Iduna – Interviewed by Brenda Bowers, July 16, 1976 and July 20, 1976.

40.   Hawks, Marvin – Interviewed by Karen Cecil Smith, June 22, 1998.

41.   Quesinberry, Iduna – Interviewed by Brenda Bowers, July 16, 1976 and July 20, 1976.

42.   Pruitt, Lackie – Interviewed by Brenda Bowers, August 10, 1976.

43.   Worrell, Wavy – Interviewed by Karen Cecil Smith, July 11, 1997.

44.   Worrell, Wavy – Interviewed by Karen Cecil Smith, July 11, 1997.

45.   Puckett, David – Interviewed by Karen Cecil Smith, September 15, 1998.

46.   Worrell, Wavy – Interviewed by Karen Cecil Smith, July 11, 1997.

47.   Worrell, Wavy – Interviewed by Karen Cecil Smith, July 11, 1997.

48.   Information provided by The American Chestnut Foundation, Bennington, VT.

49. Information provided by The American Chestnut Foundation, Bennington, VT.

50. Information provided by The American Chestnut Foundation, Bennington, VT.

51. Worrell, Wavy – Interviewed by Karen Cecil Smith, July 11, 1997.

52. Worrell, Wavy – Interviewed by Karen Cecil Smith, July 11, 1997.

53. Quesinberry, Iduna – Interviewed by Brenda Bowers, July 16, 1976 and July 20, 1976.

54. Worrell, Wavy – Interviewed by Karen Cecil Smith, July 11, 1997.

55. Worrell, Wavy – Interviewed by Brenda Bowers, July 16, 1976 and July 20, 1976.

56. Worrell, Wavy – Interviewed by Karen Cecil Smith, July 11, 1997.

57. Worrell, Wavy – Interviewed by Karen Cecil Smith, July 11, 1997.

58. Worrell, Wavy – Interviewed by Karen Cecil Smith, July 11, 1997.

59. Puckett, David – Interviewed by Karen Cecil Smith, September 15, 1998.

60. Worrell, Wavy – Interviewed by Karen Cecil Smith, July 11, 1997.

61. Worrell, Wavy – Interviewed by Karen Cecil Smith, July 11, 1997.

62. Quesinberry, Iduna – Interviewed by Brenda Bowers, July 16, 1976 and July 20, 1976.

63. Puckett, Hattie – Interviewed by Karen Cecil Smith, May 18, 1997.

64. Worrell, Wavy – Interviewed by Karen Cecil Smith, July 11, 1997.

65. Puckett, David – Interviewed by Karen Cecil Smith, September 15, 1998.

66. Puckett, Hattie – Interviewed by Karen Cecil Smith, May 18, 1997.

67. Hawks, Marvin – Interviewed by Karen Cecil Smith, June 22, 1998.

68. Bowman, Mrs. Ellis – Interviewed by Brenda Bowers, August 20, 1976.

69. Puckett, Larma – Interviewed by Karen Cecil Smith, July 16, 1998.

70. Worrell, Wavy – Interviewed by Karen Cecil Smith, July 23, 1998.

71. Quesinberry, Iduna – Interviewed by Brenda Bowers, July 16, 1976 and July 20, 1976.

72. Worrell, Wavy – Interviewed by Karen Cecil Smith, July 11, 1997.

73. Quesinberry, Iduna – Interviewed by Brenda Bowers, July 16, 1976 and July 20, 1976.

74. Hawks, Marvin – Interviewed by Karen Cecil Smith, June 22, 1998.

75. Quesinberry, Iduna – Interviewed by Brenda Bowers, July 16, 1976 and July 20, 1976.

76. Quesinberry, Iduna – Interviewed by Brenda Bowers, July 16, 1976 and July 20, 1976.

77. Bowman, Charlie – Interviewed by Brenda Bowers, July 26, 1976.

78. Hawks, Marvin – Interviewed by Karen Cecil Smith, June 22, 1998.

79. Worrell, Wavy – Interviewed by Karen Cecil Smith, July 11, 1997.

80. Quesinberry, Iduna – Interviewed by Brenda Bowers, July 16, 1976 and July 20, 1976.

81. Hawks, Marvin – Interviewed by Karen Cecil Smith, June 22, 1998.

82. Hawks, Marvin – Interviewed by Karen Cecil Smith, June 22, 1998.

83. Worrell, Wavy – Interviewed by Karen Cecil Smith, July 11, 1997.

Chapter 6 – Midwifery

1. Hawks, Marvin – Interviewed by Karen Cecil Smith, June 22, 1998.

2. Martin, Coy – Interviewed by Brenda Bowers, July 13, 1976.

3. Bowman, Mrs. Ellis – Interviewed by Brenda Bowers, August 20, 1976.

4. Worrell, Wavy – Interviewed by Karen Cecil Smith, October, 1998.

5. Martin, Coy – Interviewed by Brenda Bowers, July 13, 1976.

6. Gibson, Faith, *Contributions by the Midwives of Antiquity to the Art and Science of Modern Medicine*, www.goodnewsnet.org/practice/antiqmdw.htm

7. Gibson, *Contributions by the Midwives of Antiquity to the Art and Science of Modern Medicine*.

8. Worrell, Wavy – Interviewed by Karen Cecil Smith, July 11, 1997.

9. Puckett, Larma – Interviewed by Karen Cecil Smith, July 16, 1998.

10. Worrell, Wavy – Interviewed by Karen Cecil Smith, July 11, 1997.

11. Worrell, Wavy – Interviewed by Karen Cecil Smith, October, 1998.

12. Hawks, Foy – Interviewed by Karen Cecil Smith, April 6, 1997.

13. Hawks, Marvin – Interviewed by Karen Cecil Smith, June 22, 1998.

14. Marshall, Lottie – Interviewed by Karen Cecil Smith, July 16, 1998.

15. Puckett, Hattie – Interviewed by Karen Cecil Smith, May 18, 1997.

16. Puckett, Hattie – Interviewed by Karen Cecil Smith, Mary 18, 1997.

17. *Help for Midwives,* Bureau of Vital Statistics, Richmond, VA, 1927, pp. 1, 2, 17, 18.

18. Worrell, Wavy – Interviewed by Karen Cecil Smith, July 11, 1997.

19. Worrell, Wavy - Interviewed by Karen Cecil Smith, July 11, 1997.

20. Puckett, Larma – Interviewed by Karen Cecil Smith, July 16, 1998.

21. Worrell, Wavy – Interviewed by Karen Cecil Smith, July 11, 1997.

22. Hawks, Foy – Interviewed by Karen Cecil Smith, April 6, 1997.

23. Brady, Fanny – Interviewed by Brenda Bowers, August 3, 1976.

24. Martin, Mrs. Coy – Interviewed by Brenda Bowers, July 13, 1976.

25. Pruitt, Mrs. Raymond – Interviewed by Brenda Bowers, July 12, 1976.

26. Culler, Mrs. Dewey – Interviewed by Brenda Bowers, July 30, 1976.

27. Pruitt, Raymond – Interviewed by Brenda Bowers, July 12, 1976.

28. Martin, Coy – Interviewed by Brenda Bowers, July 13, 1976.

29. Puckett, Larma – Interviewed by Karen Cecil Smith, July 16, 1998.

30. Quesinberry, Iduna – Interviewed by Brenda Bowers, July 16, 1997 and July 20, 1976.

31. Bowman, Mrs. Ellis – Interviewed by Brenda Bowers, August 20, 1976.

32. Martin, Mrs. Coy – Interviewed by Brenda Bowers, July 13, 1976.

33. Bowman, Mrs. Ellis – Interviewed by Brenda Bowers, August 20, 1976.

34. Pruitt, Lackie – Interviewed by Brenda Bowers, August 10, 1976.

35. Davids, *The Man Who Moved A Mountain,* pp. 12, 14.

36. Davids, *The Man Who Moved A Mountain,* pp. 20, 21.

37. Willis, *Folk Lore of A Mountainous Section of Southwest Virginia, Country Living,* pp. 1-2.

38. Quesinberry, Iduna – Interviewed by Brenda Bowers, July 16, 1976 and July 20, 1976.

39. Puckett, Bell – Interviewed by Brenda Bowers, August 10, 1976.

40. Worrell, Wavy – Interviewed by Karen Cecil Smith, July 11, 1997.

41. Bowman, Charlie – Interviewed by Brenda Bowers, July 26, 1976.

42. Worrell, Wavy – Interviewed by Karen Cecil Smith, July 11, 1997.

43. Martin, Coy – Interviewed by Brenda Bowers, July 13, 1976.

44. Vass, Icy – Interviewed by Karen Cecil Smith, June 22, 1998.

45. Bowman, Mrs. Ellis – Interviewed by Brenda Bowers, August 20, 1976.

46. Puckett, Larma – Interviewed by Karen Cecil Smith, July 16, 1998.

47. Puckett, Larma – Interviewed by Karen Cecil Smith, July 16, 1998.

48. Hawks, Icy – Interviewed by Karen Cecil Smith, June 22, 1998.

49. Worrell, Wavy – Interviewed by Karen Cecil Smith, July 11, 1997.

50. Puckett, Larma – Interviewed by Karen Cecil Smith, July 16, 1998.

51. Marshall, Lottie – Interviewed by Karen Cecil Smith, July 16, 1998.

52. Willis, Ninevah J. – Interviewed by Karen Cecil Smith, June 9, 1998.

53. Spellings, Dee – Interviewed by Karen Cecil Smith, August 7, 1998.

54. Willis, Ninevah J. – Interviewed by Karen Cecil Smith, June 9, 1998.

55. Worrell, Wavy – Interviewed by Karen Cecil Smith, July 11, 1997.

56. Bowman, Mrs. Ellis – Interviewed by Brenda Bowers, August 20, 1976.

57. Puckett, Hattie – Interviewed by Karen Cecil Smith, May, 18, 1997.

58. Hawks, Marvin – Interviewed by Karen Cecil Smith, June 22, 1998.

59. Puckett, Hattie – Interviewed by Karen Cecil Smith, May, 18, 1997.

60. Hawks, Foy – Interviewed by Karen Cecil Smith, April 6, 1997.

61. Ashburn, Jesse A., *History of the Fisher's River Primitive Baptist Association,From Its Organization in 1832, to 1904*, p. 83.

62. Ashburn, *History of the Fisher's River Primitive Baptist Association From Its Organization in 1832, to 1904*, p. 85.

63. Hawks, Marvin – Interviewed by Karen Cecil Smith, June 22, 1998.

64. Worrell, Wavy – Interviewed by Karen Cecil Smith, July 11, 1997.

Chapter 7 – The Blue Ridge Parkway

1. Puckett, Hattie – Interviewed by Karen Cecil Smith, May 18, 1997.

2. *1935 It Was the Beginning of Things To Come, The Gazette,* Galax, VA, September 6, 1985, pp. 2H, 4H.

3. *1935 It Was the Beginning of Things To Come, The Gazette,* Galax, VA, September 6, 1985, pp. 2H, 4H.

4. *1935 It Was the Beginning of Things To Come, The Gazette,* Galax, VA, September 6, 1985, pp. 2H, 4H.

5. *1935 It Was the Beginning of Things To Come, The Gazette,* Galax, VA, September 6, 1985, pp. 2H, 4H.

6. Bullins, Tina, *Adventure and Hard Work Were Involved In Construction, The Gazette,* Galax, VA, September 6, 1985, p. 6P.

7. Funk, Angela, *Higgins Took Time Out From Work To Get Married, The Gazette,* Galax, VA, September 6, 1985, p. 10P.

8. Padgett, Ottie, *Hack Meredith Injured During Construction, The Gazette,* September 6, 1985, p. 14P.

9. Funk, *Fender Worked On Public Works,* p. 8P.

10. Bullins, *Handy Recalls Walking 62 Miles Backwards On the Parkway In '39,* p. 22P.

11. *Hard Work Caused Webb Problems, The Gazette,* Galax, VA, September 6, 1985, pp. 16H, 20H.

12. Funk, *James Wagoner Says Working On the Parkway Sometimes Dangerous,* p. 6P.

13. Bullins, *Handy Recalls Walking 62 Miles Backwards On the Parkway In '39,* p. 22P.

14. Padgett, Ottie, *Padgett Recalls Working Hard for 30 Cents An Hour, The Gazette*, Galax, VA, September 6, 1985, p. 20P.

15. Bullins, *Adventure and Hard Work,* p. 6P.

16. Chambers, Larry, *Hale Remembers Run Before Dynamite Exploded, The Gazette*, Galax, VA, September 6, 1985, p. 10P.

17. Funk, Angela, *Cole's Parkway Career Spans Several Decades,The Gazette*, Galax, VA, September 6, 1985, p. 18P.

18. Funk, *Cole's Parkway Career,* p. 18P.

19. Chambers, *Hale Remembers Run,* p. 10P.

20. Chambers, *Hale Remembers Run,* p. 10P.

21. Bullins, Tina, *Brothers-in-Law Worked On Parkway Together, The Gazette*, Galax, VA, September 6, 1985, p. 6H.

22. Padgett, *Hack Meredith Injured,* p. 14P.

23. Bullins, Tina, *Fortner and Father Traveled Over 30 Miles To Work, The Gazette,* Galax, VA, September 6, 1985, p. 4P.

24. Bullins, *Fortner and Father Traveled,* p. 4P.

25. Padgett, Ottie, *Parkway Provided Job For Hawks, The Gazette,* Galax, VA, September 6, 1985, p. 18H.

26. Padgett, *Parkway Provided Job,* p. 18H.

27. Bullins, *Adventure and Hard Work,* 6P.

28. Bullins, *Adventure and Hard Work,* 6P.

29. *1935 It Was the Beginning of Things To Come,* p. 4H.

30. *1935 It Was the Beginning of Things To Come,* p. 4H.

31. *1935 It Was the Beginning of Things To Come,* p. 4H.

32. Burnette, Kimberly, *The Blue Ridge Parkway and Its Effects on Local People, Mileposts and More: The Blue Ridge Parkway* by Anthropology 411: Appalachian Cultures Class, Radford University, Spring Semester, 1985, p. 21.

33. Burnette, *The Blue Ridge Parkway and Its Effect on Local People,* p. 21.

34. Burnette, *The Blue Ridge Parkway and Its Effect on Local People,* p. 22.

35. Burnette, *The Blue Ridge Parkway and Its Effect on Local People,* p. 22.

36. *Mabry Mill Is Popular Landmark, The Gazette,* Galax, VA, September 6, 1985, p. 22A.

37. Burnette, *The Blue Ridge Parkway and Its Effect on Local People*, p. 22.

38. Burnette, *The Blue Ridge Parkway and Its Effect on Local People*, p. 22.

39. Burnette, *The Blue Ridge Parkway and Its Effect on Local People*, p. 22.

40. Burnette, *The Blue Ridge Parkway and Its Effect on Local People*, p. 23.

41. Burnette, *The Blue Ridge Parkway and Its Effect on Local People*, p. 23.

42. Burnette, *The Blue Ridge Parkway and Its Effect on Local People*, p. 23.

43. Burnette, *The Blue Ridge Parkway and Its Effect on Local People*, p. 24.

44. Burnette, *The Blue Ridge Parkway and Its Effect on Local People*, p. 25.

45. Burnette, *The Blue Ridge Parkway and Its Effect on Local People*, p. 25.

46. Burnette, *The Blue Ridge Parkway and Its Effect on Local People*, p. 25.

47. Burnette, *The Blue Ridge Parkway and Its Effect on Local People*, p. 25.

48. Burnette, *The Blue Ridge Parkway and Its Effect on Local People*, p. 25.

49. Martin, Coy – Interviewed by Brenda Bowers, July 13, 1976.

50. Martin, Coy – Interviewed by Brenda Bowers, July 13, 1976.

51. Puckett, Hattie – Interviewed by Karen Cecil Smith, May 18, 1997.

52. Hawks, Marvin – Interviewed by Karen Cecil Smith, June 22, 1998.

53. Hawks, Marvin – Interviewed by Karen Cecil Smith, June 22, 1998.

Chapter 8 – Journey's End

1. Pruitt, Mrs. Lackie – Interviewed by Brenda Bowers, August 10, 1976.
2. Wigginton, Eliot, *Foxfire 2,* Anchor Books, Garden City, NY, 1973, p. 306.
3. *Home-Made Caskets, Carroll County Heritage, Vol. II,* Carroll County Genealogy Club, Hillsville, VA, p. 38.
4. Puckett, Larma – Interviewed by Karen Cecil Smith, July 16, 1998.
5. Puckett, Larma – Interviewed by Karen Cecil Smith, July 16, 1998.
6. *Home-Made Caskets, Carroll County Heritage, Vol. II,* p.38.
7. Puckett, Larma – Interviewed by Karen Cecil Smith, July 16, 1998.
8. Wigginton, *Foxfire 2,* p. 309.
9. Puckett, Larma – Interviewed by Karen Cecil Smith, July 16, 1998.
10. Hawks, Icy – Interviewed by Karen Cecil Smith, June 22, 1998.
11. Turner, H. M., *When I Am Gone, The Old School Hymnal, No.8,* J. A. Monsees, Atlanta, GA, 1942, p. 42.
12. Puckett, Larma – Interviewed by Karen Cecil Smith, July 16, 1998.
13. Hawks, Marvin – Interviewed by Karen Cecil Smith, June 22, 1998.
14. Bowman, Ellis – Interviewed by Brenda Bowers, August 20, 1976.

Epilogue

1. Citizens for Midwifery, www.cfmidwifery.org/faq.html
2. Chandrasekaran, Rajiv, *Midwife Charged in Death of Newborn Baby, The Washington Post,* May 18, 1996, p. A01,

www.gentlebirth.org/archives/mhughes.html

3. Chandrasekaran, *Midwife Charged,* p. A01.

4. Neuberger, Christine, *Two Midwives Face Charges in Death, Richmond Times Dispatch,* January 21, 1999, p. B-1; *Mom Needed Transfusion, Affidavits Say, Richmond Times Dispatch,* January 22, 1999, p. B-1.

5. www.cfmidwifery.org/faq.html

6. Medwin, Amy – Interviewed by Karen Cecil Smith, January 27, 1999.

7. *Statutory Laws,* Code of Virginia Database Legislative Information System, http://leg1.state.va.us/cgi-bin/ legp504.exe?000+cod+32.1-145

Bibliography

Books, Articles, Government Publications, Websites, Other Published Sources

Ashburn, Jesse A., *History of the Fisher's River Primitive Baptist Association, from its Organization in 1832 to 1904.*

Bowers, Brenda, *Oral History Transcriptions for Puckett Cabin, 1976.*

Burnette, Kimberly, *The Blue Ridge Parkway and Its Effects On Local People, Mileposts and More: The Blue Ridge Parkway,* by Anthropology 411: Appalachian Cultures Class, Spring Semester, Radford University, 1985. Permission given by Dr. Melinda Wagner, Radford University, Radford, VA.

Carroll County Heritage, Vol. I, Carroll County, Virginia 1842-1994, Walsworth Publishing Co., 1994.

Carroll County Heritage, Vol. II, Carroll County, Virginia, Walsworth Publishing Co., 1977.

Chandrasekaran, Rajiv, *The Washington Post,* 1996. From the website: www.gentlebirth.org/archives/mhughes.html

Citizens for Midwifery, www.cfmidwifery.org/faq.html

Clifton, Neale, *Regimental Histories of Our Ancestors – Confederate States of America – 50th Virginia Infantry,* http://www.pilot.infi.net/~nkcliftn/csaregim.htm

Croteau, Maureen and Worcester, Wayne, *The Essential Researcher,* Harper Collins Publishers, New York, NY, 1993.

Dan River District, VA Census 1870, 1880.

Davids, Richard C., *The Man Who Moved A Mountain*, Fortress Press, Philadelphia, PA, 1970.

Gibson, Faith, *Contributions by the Midwives of Antiquity to the Art and Science of Modern Medicine*, www.goodnewsnet.org/practice/antiqmdw.htm

Help for Midwives, Bureau of Vital Statistics, Richmond, VA, 1927 Reprint.

History of the American Chestnut, The American Chestnut Story, The American Chestnut Foundation, Bennington, VT. http://chestnut.acf.org/history.html

Kunz, Jeffrey R. M. and Finkel, Asher, Jr., *The American Medical Association Family Medical Guide*, Random House, Inc., New York, 1987.

Land Office Patents and Grants, Virginia Counties of Amherst, Grayson, and Patrick for years 1801, 1802, 1806, 1836, 1851, 1857, 1877.

Lonn, Ella, *Desertion During the Civil War*, The American Historical Association, Gloucester, Mass., 1982. Reprinted by permission of Appleton-Century-Crofts, Inc., 1966.

Neuberger, Christine, *Richmond Times-Dispatch*, 1999.

Patrick County, VA Census, 1860.

Pilson, Betty A. and Baughan, Barbara C., *Patrick County, Virginia Birth Records 1853-1869, Patrick County; Patrick County, Virginia Birth Records 1870-1880; Virginia Death Records 1868, 1869, & 1871-1896,* 1997.

Ray, Delia, *Behind the Blue and Gray,* Lodestar Books, Laing Communications, Inc., Bellevue, WA, 1991.

Republican Newspaper, Yadkinville, NC, Article titled *A Remarkable Woman,* which included a letter to the editor from Rev. C. C. Haymore, 1900.

Smith, May Belle T., *The Puckett Family Genealogy – 1998.*

Statutory Laws, Code of Virginia Database Legislative Information System,
http://leg1.state.va.us/cgi-bin/legp504.exe?000+cpd+32.1-145

Strait, Alan, *Brother Against Brother,* http://members.tripod.com/~ALZWIRED/cwone

Surry County, NC Census 1850, 1860.

Surry County, NC Marriages, 1779-1868.

The Gazette Newspaper, *1935 Was the Beginning of Things to Come,* Galax, VA, 1985. Permission given by the editor to quote from the entire supplement on the construction of the Blue Ridge Parkway in Virginia.

The History Place – U. S. Civil War 1861-1865, http://wwww.historyplace.com/civilwar/

Turner, H. M., *When I Am Gone,* from *The Old School Hymnal No. 8,* Atlanta, GA, J. A. Monsees, 1942. Permission given by Old School Hymnal Company, Ellenwood, GA.

Walker, Gary C., *The War In Southwest Virginia 1861-65,* A & W Enterprise, Roanoke, VA, 1985.

Wigginton, Eliot, *Foxfire 2,* Anchor Books, Garden City, NY, 1973.

Willis, Ninevah J., *Folk Lore of a Mountainous Section of Southwest Virginia, Typical Mountain People, Country Living,* private unpublished collection held by the Hillsville Historical Society, Hillsville, VA.

CPSIA information can be obtained
at www.ICGtesting.com
Printed in the USA
LVOW08s0258110317
526859LV00003B/4/P